D1615802

ALLEN COUNTY PUBLIC LIBRARY
FORT WAYNE, INDIANA 46802

You may return this book to any agency, branch,

or bookmobile of the Allen County Public Library.

DEMCO

Yoga

Exercises

For Every Body

By **Ruth Bender**

Phys. Ed. and Yoga Instructor

Photographs by Alan Nenonen and Werner Bender

RUBEN PUBLISHING
Avon, Connecticut

Yoga For Every Body

© Copyright, 1975 by

RUTH BENDER

Third Printing

All Rights Reserved

ISBN 0-917434-00-5

Typesetting by Belle Typesetting Co., Avon, Connecticut
Printed by Van Way-Webco, New Britain, Connecticut

RUBEN PUBLISHING
P.O. Box 414
Avon, Connecticut 06001

7123939

INTRODUCTION:

Yoga is for people of all ages. Practiced regularly, it will help one to live a longer, healthier, happier and more productive life.

This book is a logical, common sense approach to Yoga exercise. Contraindications to specific movements are noted and no unsubstantiated claims are made. It shows the expertise that Mrs. Bender has developed over thirty-five years of Yoga experience.

Mrs. Bender is a teacher's teacher, having trained many Yoga teachers over the years. Her techniques and care in not forcing the body beyond its capabilities make it possible for any one, no matter how stiff and inflexible he may be, to get started in Yoga and to advance within his own physical parameters.

Thousands of people have benefited from the teachings of this most remarkable lady. I am certain this book will enable many more to experience the many advantages a logical, systematic Yoga program has to offer.

Dr. Dale E. Turner
Natureopathic Physician

3

FOREWORD

The idea to write this book came from my students. Very often one or another came to me after being in my class for weeks or months and suggested that I should write down the way I worked them up slowly to the more advanced Yoga postures. They had started practicing Yoga by trying to learn it from a book and had gotten very discouraged. Unfortunately all Yoga books start much too advanced for the bad physical condition of most people.

Today people are getting more and more interested in physical fitness and health and are looking for something which can bring their weak, flabby and stiff muscles to strength, tone and flexibility. For most of them calisthenics, slimnastics, modern dance or ballet are too strenuous and they shy away from it. But Yoga exercises taught the right way are the answer. They start gently and work gradually on every part of the body. This is the best beginning for people who have not done any physical activity for years.

Let's look for a moment at the inside of our body. There are bones, muscles and organs, but the important part is the connective tissue that holds it all together. Through lack of exercise and the aging process this tissue gets shortened. The longer you have lived without doing regular exercises, the more slowly and carefully you have to start to stretch these shortened connective tissues. Most Yoga exercises are gentle stretches, then holding the stretch without feeling any strain (never any bouncing). This way you will get flexible again without muscle pain.

More and more physical education departments at Universities and coaches are recognizing the benefits of the gentle stretching exercise in physical conditioning. The systematic stretching of all parts of the body also prevents pain and injury.

If you are over twenty, you should do a daily stretching routine to keep your connective tissues in good stretchable condition. Quite a number of football teams are now doing stretches (Yoga exercises) instead of calisthenics. (They are not loose enough yet to call the stretches Yoga exercises.)

5

From my thirty-five years of experience in teaching physical education and Yoga to all ages and to all physical conditions, I have developed this gentle, progressing system, which first uses very easy stretching movements to get the stiff and tight muscles and connective tissues flexible again. When they are brought to good condition and the body is ready, then step by step the more advanced Yoga Postures are introduced. The sequence in which the exercises are practiced is very important; every part of the body should get moved and stretched systematically in each session (ideally 40 to 50 minutes long).

To make it easy for students and teachers to work with this book, I bring a 10 week course with step by step progression. Each working session is complete so that looking back and forth in the book is unnecessary. To follow the directions precisely is of importance. In the whole Yoga exercise system there is not one movement or exercise without a reason or a purpose. Only in this way can you get all the benefits from this beautiful exercise system.

It works not only on your muscles and your connective tissues but also brings your internal organs and your glandular system to good working order. It also increases the blood circulation throughout your body and relaxes your nervous system. It brings your body into good physical condition, to good health, firms up, slims down, relaxes, gets rid of tension and makes you feel good all over and all under. It can help you to overcome small health problems, but if you have bigger problems, see your doctor. Yoga exercises are not a cure-all and all the health benefits many Yoga books mention are exaggerated.

I think I have been very lucky to have studied with one of the best Yoga teachers in Europe, Selvarajan Yesudian, a native of India, who conducts a Yoga School in Zuerich, Switzerland. He has a medical background and his approach and emphasis is more on the therapeutic and preventive effect of the Yoga Postures. He does not put so much value on the acrobatic side, which unfortunately quite a number of other Yoga teachers from India prefer to teach. These teachers who start too advanced, can interest only the students who are flexible. The average person who needs the gentle approach gets turned off and thinks Yoga exercises are not for his stiff and tense body. But these are the people needing it most. They are the ones I like to teach how to bring their bodies to good condition, making them feel good and alive and giving them a good healthy and flexible body.

One of the beautiful effects is also that most people start to enjoy other activities again. Everything you do, you will do better after practicing Yoga exercises for a while regularly. Your golf score will get better. You will play better tennis. Even modern dancers get more flexible. Yoga does not interfere with other activities; it helps you to enjoy them more.

Ruth Bender received her degree in physical education from the University of Munich, Germany. She has studied Yoga with Selvarajan Yesudian in Zurich, Switzerland for 2 years and spent the summer of 1968 in Yesudian's Summer School in Ponte Tresa, Switzerland.

She has taught Yoga Exercises to literally thousands of students. Presently she conducts classes in West Hartford, Farmington, and Avon, Connecticut.

She is also training interested and qualified students to teach Yoga Exercises with emphasis on how to teach beginners and people in bad physical condition. The teacher's training course is held in Farmington, Connecticut. Interested students come from all parts of this country and Canada to learn her gentle and progressive way of teaching. Many more people will get the benefits of this gentle stretching method through this book.

Ruth Bender's educational background and the study at the Yoga School in Zurich helped her to create this graduated method to gently get people into better condition and to make them more flexible.

GUIDELINES FOR THE PRACTICE OF YOGA EXERCISES.

Wear comfortable, not restricting clothes. Sweatpants and sweatshirt with socks are perfect for everybody, especially if the temperature in the room you are practicing in is under 70 degrees. If it is warmer in the room, leotards and tights for women, shorts and shirt for men are all right. The important factor is that you feel comfortable and that your muscles are kept warm; you should never get a cold or chilly feeling.

The exercise room should be comfortably warm; ideally 70-72 degrees. It also should be well ventilated. Fresh air, essential for the Yoga breathing exercises and the Yoga movements and postures, is very necessary for you all the time.

The exercises should be done on a pad or carpet, thick enough so that you cannot feel the bones of your spine when you roll back and forth on them.

The movements should be done slowly and carefully in a very relaxed manner. If you have had any back problems, check with your doctor before starting with the Yoga exercises. But please take along this book or the record "Yoga For Beginners," so that he can see what kind of exercises you are going to do. Unfortunately many people and many medical doctors think about headstand, lotusseat and pretzel-like postures when they hear Yoga exercises mentioned. But there are many other exercises which can especially benefit every part of your body. Some of the exercises are even prescribed by orthopedic doctors for their patients, and neither of them know that they are also Yoga exercises.

The best time to practice is before lunch or before dinner. In the morning your body is still stiff from sleeping and doing the exercises right after getting up does not feel very good. If it is the only convenient time for you to do them, the best way would be to do something around the house first to limber up your body or to take a hot shower and then do your exercises. You may not be able to stretch as well as in the late afternoon or evening but you will get the same benefits out of the exercises.

Do not practice your exercises shortly after eating. Wait at least one hour after a light meal, 3-4 hours after a heavier meal. It would also be a good idea to take the phone off the hook, when you start practicing, because jumping up suddenly during one of the exercises, could easily strain a muscle.

During the movements, close your eyes (in the beginning only during the lying exercises) and feel your muscles move, become aware of what is going on inside of your body, get to know your body. You will soon know how far you can stretch or bend without straining, but you will also feel how the point of strain goes farther and farther away and your body gets more and more flexible with every practice session. In time you will be able to hold the postures easily and relaxed. Also you will feel how the blood circulation is increasing in the different parts of your body during the Yoga postures.

Yoga exercises are not competitive, you are only working for yourself. So if you are practicing in a Yoga class, don't look at your neighbor, just close your eyes and watch your body inside. Everybody is built differently, and in Yoga, more than in any other exercise system, this plays a very important role. Some people just cannot do certain exercises because of the way their bodies are built. Any good teacher can see that, and will not ask these persons to do some exercises they could not do without hurting themselves.

If you are pregnant, check with your doctor. Take the book along and show him the exercises you are going to do. If there are no complications most of the exercises will benefit you. Some of them you should not do, or should do them only very gently, so watch the instructions. I will point out the ones which are not beneficial at that time.

INTRODUCTION TO YOUR FIRST YOGA LESSON.

Sit in your most comfortable chair and read the introduction and description of your first Yoga session. I would like to tell you what we are going to do during the first class and why we will do it.

If you are a teacher and are teaching the first class, let your students lie down and tell them what you are going to teach them during the first session.

Before you start with the Yoga exercises lie down for a few minutes and relax. Let your body go completely limp, close your eyes and find the most comfortable position. Lie on the floor and your carpet or pad, do not lie on a mattress. If you don't feel comfortable stretched out, then bend your knees, put your feet on the mat and gently press your back down. If you have back problems, swayback, or if you are pregnant, you will feel better in this position. Your back muscles can relax better this way. Just let yourself go and relax. The more relaxed you are the more easily you can do the following movements.

After relaxing this way for about 5 minutes roll on your right side, put your elbow down and sit up slowly over your right side.

Sitting up over your right side is important in the beginning of your Yoga career: During one session you will lie down and sit up quite a number of times. If you get up straight to a sitting position every time, your weak abdominal muscles would hurt you the next day. Coming up over your right side will work your muscles but not strain them. Any muscle which gets strained will get weaker, not stronger. To come up over your right side also helps to keep your heart muscle relaxed.

Then stand up slowly and now we are going to start with the Warm-up exercises.

The Warm-up Exercises are the most important part of any exercise system; but they are especially important before the slowly done Yoga exercises. If a cold and stiff muscle gets stretched, it can very easily get strained or even injured. Through the warm-ups the blood will circulate well in the muscle tissue and make them soft and pliable, so stretching cannot harm them. Also the joints have to be warmed up through gentle relaxed movements, done not too fast and not too slowly; do them in a rather sloppy, relaxed way. There are two kinds of warm-ups: The active and the passive kind. The active warm-up is through relaxed, fairly fast movements, involving every part of the body step by step.

The passive warm-up is accomplished through hot bath, hot shower, Sauna or steam bath.

Before Yoga exercises I recommend the active warm-up, which also adds to the physical fitness and has a slimming and firming-up effect.

Also before any other sport activity you can or should do this easy warm-up. After a few days you will know the movements by heart. Do them before playing tennis, before swimming, jogging, playing golf. You will be surprised how much easier you can move and the important thing you will prevent injury to your muscles or joints.

THE 6 WARM-UP EXERCISES.

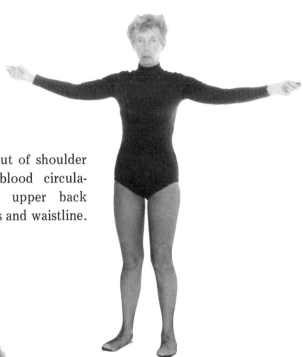

ARM SWINGING.

Gets stiffness out of shoulder joints, increases blood circulation, stretches upper back muscles, slims hips and waistline.

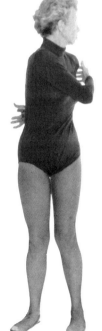

1. Put your feet comfortably apart.
2. Stretch your arms out to the sides.
3. Swing your arms relaxed around your body.
4. Turn your body gently while looking back.

About 10 X

(If you should start feeling dizzy, keep looking straight ahead.)

1ST WEEK.

KNEE RAISING.

Loosens up the knee and hip joints, gives the abdominal organs a gentle massage.

1. Put your feet together.
2. Raise your right knee up, clasp your hands around it.
3. Put your right foot down. Repeat with your left leg.

About 10 X

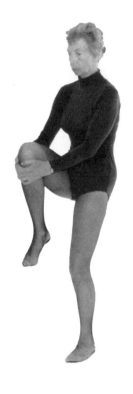

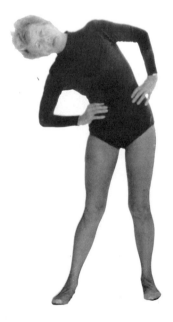

SIDE BEND.

Gently stretches the muscles along the sides of the spine and the sides of your body.

1. Put your feet comfortably apart.
2. Put your hands to your hips.
3. Bend your body gently to your right side.
4. Bend your body gently to your left side.

3 X each side.

ARM CIRCLES.

Loosens up the shoulder joints and makes the blood circulate better. Swing backwards (like swimming the back crawl). Important for women to strengthen the muscles in the chest to give a beautiful bustline. Start with one arm alone.

1. Put your feet together.
2. Stretch your right arm up.
3. Let it fall back and swing it around.
4. Turn your body slightly to your right.
   Swing relaxed and easy.

10 X

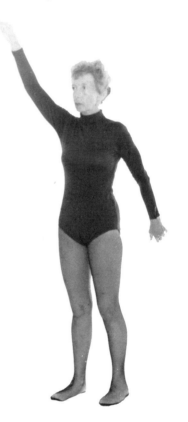

Do the same with your left arm.

If you can swing each arm alone easily and relaxed, try to do it with both arms.

1. Stretch one arm forward, one back.
2. Swing your arms backwards and around.

10 X

ARM MOVEMENTS FOR PEOPLE WITH BURSITIS.

If you have bursitis and cannot do the arm circles without pain, then practice the following arm movements until the pain is gone when raising the arm over shoulder height.

PENDULUM.

1. Put your feet comfortably apart.
2. Bend forward, put your left hand on left knee.
3. Let right arm gently swing from side to side.
   Repeat with left arm.
   About 20 X each arm

When this movement feels comfortable, keep the same position and make small circles with each arm.
About 20 X

If you don't feel any discomfort with the circles make small figure eights with each arm.
About 20 X

Do these movements several times during the day. The important task is to increase the blood circulation in the shoulders. Be careful with the use of cortisone.

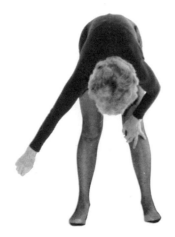 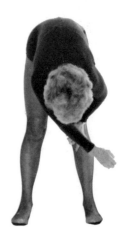

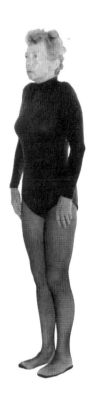

SHOULDER ROLLING.

Loosens up the muscles in shoulders and neck, strengthens the bust muscles, gives good bustline.
1. Keep your feet slightly apart.
2. Keep your arms hanging relaxed at your sides.
3. Draw your shoulders up, move them back, down and around, gently and slowly.

5 X

SQUATTING DOWN.

Moves the knee joints and makes them more flexible. Do this exercise very slowly and carefully. Don't go all the way down, only as far as you can without feeling any strain. The knee joints are the first ones to stiffen up if you don't move them enough.

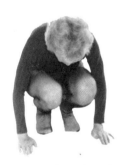

1. Put your feet comfortably apart.
2. Bend your knees slowly.
3. If you can, put your hands down on the mat.
4. Put more weight on your hands than on your knees.
5. Come up slowly.

4 X

Deep kneebends can be harmful if you do them fast or if you stay down putting all your weight on your knees. Our knees are built to be bent, but through our sedentary way of life we do not use our knees enough and they stiffen up fast. Through these gentle kneebends we bring them back to good condition and flexibility.

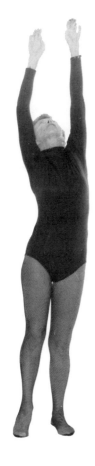

STRETCHING UP.

Stretches every muscle in your body from toes to fingertips. After warming up all the muscles in your body we now do a beautiful stretch.

1. Put your feet comfortably apart.
2. Raise your arms over your head.
3. Stretch your right side up.
4. Stretch your left side up.
   Repeat 2 X
5. Then completely relaxed, bend over. Keep your knees slightly bent during the forward bend and keep them also bent during the coming up movement. This is important, it avoids any strain on your lower back.
   Do the whole stretch 2 X

Caution: Any woman pregnant during the first three months should not do this stretching exercise.

These are the warm-up exercises, which should be done at the beginning of every Yoga session or before any other activity. A tip for the Yoga Teacher: Watching the beginners during the warm-ups can tell to a certain degree in what condition the students are, how their coordination is working, how tense or relaxed they are, how their comprehension and observation is working.

A student arriving late for class should always do the warm-ups first before joining in the activity of the class. Since the warm-ups are always done in the same sequence, the student will know them by heart after a few sessions.

But if the whole class does the warm-ups together, the teacher should lead them. If the students do them without a leader, they do not do them properly and often enough.

1ST WEEK.

THE YOGA EXERCISES OF THE FIRST SESSION.

After the warm-ups when the blood circulates well in your body, you can start with your first Yoga exercises. They work step by step through your whole body, starting with strengthening the muscles in your feet and legs. Your tiny, or not so tiny feet, have to carry your whole body. If the muscles in your feet and legs are not strong enough to carry your body properly, your back muscles have to do more work and suffer. To strengthen the foot and leg muscles, we are going to do balancing exercises.

After that we strengthen and stretch the muscles in your thighs, hips, shoulders, legs, back, stomach and neck.

Try to do every movement as relaxed and sloppy as possible. Don't work hard! Your muscles are moving and are getting stronger even when you do it relaxed and this way they don't get strained. We never work hard in Yoga, we never hurry and we never force anything. There are some muscles in your body you have not used for a long time. Our bodies are built to be moved, but in our sedentary way of life, we don't use them enough. During the Yoga exercises we will get to these stiff, tight muscles and connective tissues, but you have to move very gently. You look and watch inside your body and feel how far you can go without feeling any strain or pain. If you should feel any pain during any of the exercises, do this movement especially gently. If the pain should persist, talk to your doctor about it.

We start with very gentle movements to loosen up and to stretch the muscles and tendons. Each lesson should be practiced for one week. Then when you have practiced regularly, your body and muscles will be ready for the next slightly more advanced version of some of the exercises. Every movement we do has several versions, from the most gentle and easiest, to the most advanced. Whenever your body is ready, the more advanced exercises will be introduced. Since I cannot watch you personally like the students in my classes, I have to ask you not to go on to the exercises of the next week, if you cannot do the exercises from the preceding week easily and relaxed. You have to be patient and watch your body. Only then can

19

you get the benefits of this beautiful therapeutic and preventive exercise system.

Try to do every exercise slowly from the beginning to the end. Think about a slow motion scene on television, how it gently and slowly moves and swings. This way you will feel immediately when an uncomfortable feeling approaches and this is the point you should stop and not go farther with the stretch. If you feel a strain, you already have gone too far. If you watch yourself carefully you will observe that week by week the point of this uncomfortable feeling will go farther and farther away. That means your connective tissues are getting more and more stretched and flexible.

FIRST BALANCING EXERCISE.

Strengthens the muscles in feet and legs. Helps you to concentrate.

1. Stand on your right foot.
2. Raise your arms slightly at your sides.
3. Lift your left foot up.
4. Put your knees together.
5. Concentrate on a spot 4-5 feet in front of you.

Hold to the count of 10.

Relax your legs by gently shaking them.

Repeat on left foot.

You can feel how the muscles in your foot work to keep you balanced; this strengthens these muscles and the muscles in your leg.

If you have trouble balancing freely, hold on to the wall or to a chair until the foot muscles get stronger.

Do not balance on a soft surface (foam rubber) or in a room with dimmed lights.

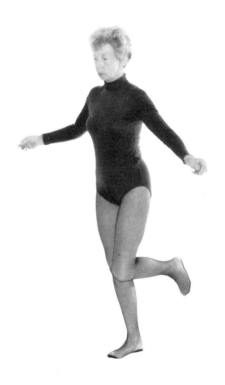

WIDE KNEE BEND AND SHIFT.

Stretches and strengthens the muscles in your legs. Firms up and slims down inner thighs. Makes knees and ankles more flexible.

1. Put your feet wider apart than is comfortable.
2. Keep feet parallel, toes pointing straight ahead.
3. Bend your right knee, keep left leg stretched.
4. Come up slowly and bend your left knee.

5 X

5. Then stay down and shift over from side to side. Keep your feet flat on the mat.

5 X

You should feel a gentle stretch in the inside of your stretched leg. If you do not feel this stretch, widen your step a few inches or bend your knee a little bit more.

A marvelous strengthening exercise for skiers, joggers, hikers and swimmers.

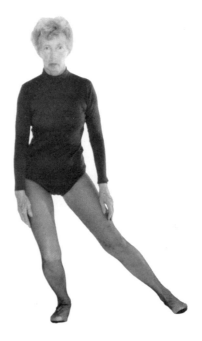

TRIANGLE POSTURE.

Slims down and firms up thighs, hips, waistline and upper body around the area behind the shoulders. Strengthens and stretches the muscles on the sides.

1. Put your feet comfortably apart.
2. Raise your arms, palms up, to shoulder height.
3. Turn right hand around, bend down to your right side.
4. Put your hand to the outside of your knee.
5. Bring your left arm closer to your head until you feel a slight stretch along your side.
6. Slowly raise your body up, turn your hands around.
7. Bend down to your left side.
8. Put your hand to the outside of your knee.
9. Bring your right arm closer to your head until you feel this gentle stretch along your side again.
10. Slowly raise your body up.

Don't bend forward during this movement, support yourself with a good hold on the outside of your knee. Feel a gentle stretch along your side, not a *strain. Don't hold* the position yet. Relax your legs, relax your shoulders.

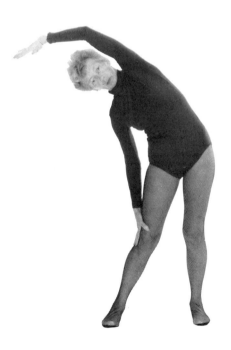

1ST WEEK.

HIPROLLS.

To relax the muscles we just stretched during the Triangle Posture. Slims down hips and waistline if you do it often and long enough.

1. Put your feet comfortably apart.
2. Put your hands to your hips.
3. Roll your hips around gently.

10 X in each direction.

Don't move upper body, just your hips should move. Do it easily, relaxed, and *slowly*.

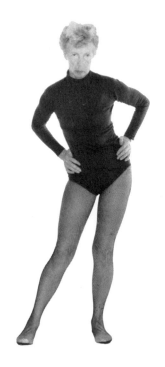

And now lie down in the most comfortable position and *relax*.

1ST WEEK.

We will always do all standing exercises first, then the lying and sitting exercises.

Between the lying and sitting exercises will be the relaxing periods, short or long depending on the nature of the preceding exercise. The relaxing is necessary to give your muscles time to recover, to collect new strength for the next exercise.

So just lie there as lazily and relaxed as possible. Close your eyes and try to relax every muscle in your body.

Some people who are not used to lying flat may feel slightly dizzy. If this should happen, take a small pillow and put it under your head. After a few weeks of practicing Yoga you will know how much relaxing time your muscles need. It is important not to lie down too long; otherwise the muscles could stiffen up again. You should feel comfortable during the relaxing time; the room should be warm. If you feel cold, put on sweatpants and sweatshirt. These are fleece-lined cotton pants and shirts available in department stores, in men's clothing or in the sports department. They come mostly in gray, but the inside is off-white. Turn them inside out and tie-dye them your favorite color. They look cute and keep your muscles warm.

After a short relaxing period, we start now with the lying exercises, which work on strengthening and relaxing your back and abdominal muscles.

1ST WEEK.

LEG RAISING.

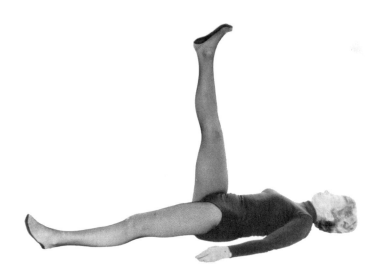

Strengthens back and abdominal muscles, firms up legs, hips, buttocks and tummy. Stretches hamstring muscles.

1. Lie on your back completely relaxed.
2. Raise your right leg slowly while inhaling.
3. Lower your right leg slowly while exhaling.
4. Raise your left leg slowly while inhaling.
5. Lower your left leg slowly while exhaling.

2 X

BOTH LEGS RAISING.

1. *Put your hands under your buttocks, palms down.*
2. Raise both legs slowly while inhaling.
3. Lower both legs slowly while exhaling.

   Not for pregnant women.

2 X

R e l a x.

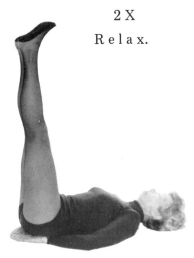

Try to do these movements relaxed, don't point your toes. If you have a back problem or especially weak back muscles, keep the lower leg bent, foot on the mat. Also good for swayback. The hands under the buttocks are an absolute must to avoid any strain of the lower back. Whenever we raise both legs or lower both legs down, the hands should be under the buttocks. The back muscles are the weakest muscles in every human being today because we don't work enough physically to keep these muscles in good condition. With these exercises we would like to strengthen the back muscles without straining them. Raising or lowering both legs without the hands under the buttocks would strain them and cause back problems. Besides that, it would tense the abdominal muscles and this results in a big tummy, just what we would like to avoid.

If you should have a slight touch of arthritis in your hands and it causes pain, then bring a towel, fold it together 8 times and put it under your buttocks.

1ST WEEK.

KNEE AND HEAD RAISING.

Relaxes the muscles in the abdominal area.

Stretches the muscles and the connective tissue in your back and neck. Stretches the muscles in your upper leg.

1. Raise your arms over your head while inhaling — s t r e t c h.
2. Bring your right knee up to your chest, press it down — exhale.

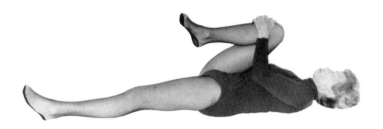

3. Gently raise your head toward your knee — inhale.
4. Put your head down — exhale (feel your neck muscles relax).
5. Stretch your leg down, your arms up — inhale — s t r e t c h.
6. Bring your left knee up to your chest, press it down — exhale.
7. Gently raise your head toward your knee — inhale.
8. Put your head down — exhale.
9. Stretch your leg down, your arms up — inhale — s t r e t c h.
10. Bring your arms down — exhale and r e l a x.

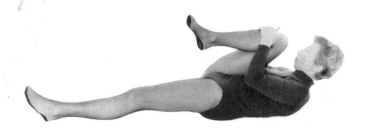

This is one of the best exercises to relax and to strengthen your back, to relieve and to prevent back problems. Done every day regularly, it will work wonders. Do it slowly with your eyes closed and watch your body inside. Doing the exercise in two stages — first

28

pressing the knee down and then raising the head — has the purpose of stretching the muscles in the back of the upper leg and thus prepares these muscles for another Yoga exercise which will be introduced in a few weeks.

When you stretch the whole body, always *stretch your heels* never your toes; you could easily get a cramp, especially when you stretch in the morning after waking up.

RAISING BOTH KNEES.

Relaxes back and abdominal muscles. Good position for a tired or strained back.

1. Raise your arms over your head while inhaling — s t r e t c h.
2. Bring both knees up to your chest *(slide feet over mat)*. Put your hands on your knees, press them down — exhale.
3. Hold this position, but relieve the pressure on your knees.
4. Breathe relaxed and consciously relax your back, relax your shoulders, relax your arms.
5. *Then put your feet on the mat first,* stretch your legs down, your arms up while inhaling — s t r e t c h your whole body
6. Put your arms down — exhale and r e l a x.

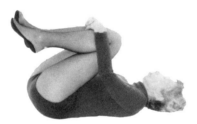

This position is also called the "wind relieving pose": If you get a little annoying pain in your intestines after eating cabbage or onions, get into this position and hold it. After about 1 minute you will get relief. But do it in the privacy of your bedroom.

Putting your feet down first, when you come out of this exercise is important, because it keeps your back down on the mat, since your hands are not under your buttocks but stretched up over your head.

NECK RELAXING MOVEMENTS.

Relieves tension in the neck and upper back, can relieve tension headache.

1. Sit in cross-legged position, try to sit straight.
   (If you feel uncomfortable in this position, then sit on a chair, but keep your back straight).
2. Slowly bring your head forward, chin to chest.
3. Then slowly raise it up and bring it back as far as you can without any strain.

3 X

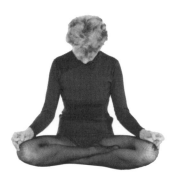 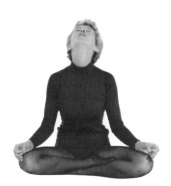

1. Turn your head to your right side — slowly.
2. Turn your head to your left side.

3 X

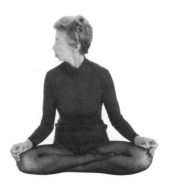 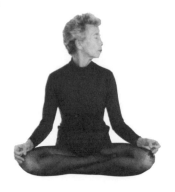

1ST WEEK.

1. Gently tilt your head to your right shoulder.
2. Slowly raise it up and tilt to your left shoulder.

3 X

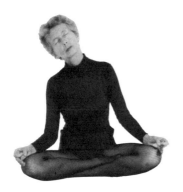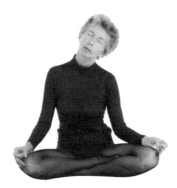

Don't move your body, only your head when you do these 3 head movements. Do them very slowly, close your eyes and feel what is going on inside.

These neck movements are very important, they relax the muscles of your upper back and neck, relieve tension and prepare and limber up your neck muscles for the Yoga exercises which follow.

These 3 neck movements should be done every morning and several times during the day, but only when the body is warm, never with cold muscles. Keep your neck warm at all times. If you had a neck injury, whiplash or arthritis, wear turtleneck sweaters (especially at night).

Some doctors call these 3 movements the "Yes, No and Maybe Exercises." But make it a very slow Yes, No and Maybe.

People with a long neck, should put their hands around the neck when they do these movements the first few weeks until the muscles are stronger.

Do not do any circles with your head. It puts too much strain on the neck muscles and the facettes of the vertebrae, and is not recommended.

ROCK AND ROLL.

After limbering up the neck, let's limber up your back with the Rock and Roll exercise. It gives your spine a gentle massage. It also massages the muscles in your back and has a calming effect on your nervous system which is built-in in your spinal column. It strengthens your abdominal muscles and prepares your body for the next exercise and others which follow in the next few weeks and months.

Caution: You should have a good padding on the floor. You should not feel the bones in your back when rolling over them. So try it first very gently. If you feel your bones even slightly, the padding is not thick enough. Put another piece of carpet or a blanket on top of it.

1. Sit up, bend your knees, feet on the mat.
2. Clasp your hands gently together under your knees.
3. Put your chin to your chest to keep your back round.
4. Swing your legs gently up and roll back to your shoulder blades.
5. Swing your legs down and roll up — feet on mat. Do it again and again, relaxed and easy.

8-10 X

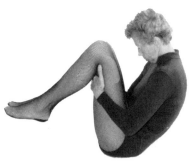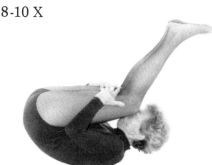

Lie down and relax.

If you have trouble rolling up during the Rock and Roll, swing your legs down a little bit faster. Your legswing should bring you up. Don't try to come up with your stomach muscles alone as that could strain them. If you should get a slight cramp in your stomach muscles, lie down and stretch.

During the Rock and Roll your head should not touch the mat, keep your back round, otherwise you will have trouble coming up.

1ST WEEK.

To keep your chin to your chest is also a safety precaution, so you do not roll over too far, your feet should not touch the floor behind your head. A beginners neck is not flexible enough to go that far back.

THE HALF SHOULDERSTAND.

Increases the blood circulation in neck and every part of the head. Prevents wrinkles in face. Increases oxygenation of brain cells. Helps to better varicose veins.

1. Lying on your back, put hands under buttocks, starting with palms down.
2. Slowly raise both legs and your hips, support them with your hands, elbows on the mat close to the body.
3. Hold this position for a few seconds. Legs in about 45° angle.
4. To come down: first lower your legs slightly farther over your head.
5. Put your hands on the mat close together.
6. *Bend your knees* and slowly roll your back down, bring your hips down and stretch your legs down. Relax.

2 X

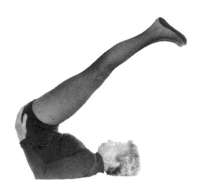

If you have trouble raising your hips slowly then start with swinging your legs up faster. If that should not work yet, start in the sitting position of the "Rock and Roll" with your knees bent, roll back and when you feel your hips coming up, stretch your legs and hold on to your hips. Even if you can only hold the position for a second or two, you will get the feeling for the position. If it still should not work, keep practicing the "Leg Raising" exercise and the "Rock and Roll" until your abdominal and back muscles are strong enough to raise your hips up. Do not do Sit-ups.

The Half Shoulderstand is one of the most beneficial exercises in the Yoga exercise system. It increases in a gentle way the blood circulation in every organ of the head and even people with high blood pressure can do it. Your face will get rosy after a few seconds, the complexion will get better after regular practice. The blood will circulate better in your eyes, ears, scalp and especially in your brain. And this is very important, because the brain needs 12 times more oxygen than any other part of the body. Through the increased blood circulation and later with the special breathing in this position, we bring more oxygen to the brain. The brain will work better, the memory will be improved, comprehension gets better and you will not get tired so easily. Experience shows that children had better test results after practicing this exercise than the group which did not practice it.

You also can feel the benefits if you are tired but still have some important work to do, or have to drive. Go into the Half Shoulderstand, holding it as long as you can easily and relaxed, and you will be surprised how fresh you will feel.

The half shoulderstand also brings the abdominal organs in a reversed position. Good for tilted uterus and weak bladder; the pressure on the bladder is relieved. If you have the problem that you have to go to the bathroom one or two or even more times at night, then it can be beneficial to do the half shoulderstand in bed just before you want to go to sleep. It is not as comfortable to do as on the mat, because the bed is too soft. But the important thing is to get the abdominal organs into the inverted position, holding it as long as comfortable. Go down very slowly. Don't sit up again, but lie in your favorite sleeping position and have a good uninterrupted sleep.

BRIDGE POSTURE.

Now we are going into the Bridge Posture to bend the spine in the opposite direction from the Half Shoulderstand.

1. Lie on your back, arms relaxed alongside your body.
2. Bend your knees, put your feet flat on the mat close to your body, about one foot apart.
3. Slowly raise your hips while inhaling.
4. Slowly lower your hips while exhaling — press your back down gently and draw your tummy in.

3 X

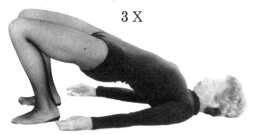

During the exercise close your eyes and watch what is going on inside your body. Watch your muscles. Only go as high up as you can without feeling any strain in your back — you can feel a slight stretch in your upper legs. Your shoulders should stay on the mat. Slowly let your spine roll up and slowly let your spine roll down. Feel every vertebra touching down. Direct your consciousness to your spine.

BENEFITS OF THE BRIDGE POSTURE.

The spine is stretched in the opposite direction from the Half Shoulderstand. The muscles and the connective tissues of the abdominal wall are stretched and the muscles of the lower back get strengthened. The abdominal organs are put into the right position. It helps to put a tilted uterus into the right position and will relieve cramps during the period, when practiced faithfully every day during the weeks between the periods. In many cases it will relieve back problems by strengthening and relaxing the back muscles. Done regularly it will prevent back problems. Caution: If pregnant, do this exercise very gently.

1ST WEEK.

THE RELAXING POSTURE.

The last exercise in each Yoga class is the Corpse Posture. I don't like this name and call it Relaxing Posture.

Just lie there and relax completely, lie as comfortably as possible. If you feel better relaxed with your knees bent, feet on the mat or with one knee bent, then lie this way. You should feel as relaxed as possible without tension.

Close your eyes and concentrate on the parts of your body I am going to mention. We start with your feet and go through every part of the body. Try to relax each part consciously by thinking about it. Feel yourself into the different parts of your body.

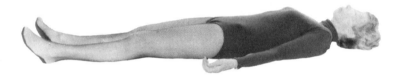

Relax your legs,
Relax your feet,
Relax your toes,
Relax your calves,
Relax your thighs,
Relax your stomach,
Relax your chest,
Relax your shoulders,
Relax your arms,
Relax your hands,
Relax your fingers,
Relax your neck,
Relax your head,
Relax your face,
Relax your mouth,
Relax your teeth,
Relax every muscle in your back,
Relax your whole body,
Relax completely.

1ST WEEK.

Find any tense spot in your body and relax it.

Now relax for about 10 minutes, but only if the room is warm and you feel comfortable. You cannot relax if the body gets cold or your feet get cold.

After about 10 minutes raise your arms over your head and stretch your whole body, then roll on your left side and stretch, roll on your right side and stretch, sit up over your right side.

Thank you, see you tomorrow.

During the Yoga session we try to work with every muscle in your body. We stretch the muscles and relax them. At the end of the session you really can feel how relaxed your muscles became. If you have not gotten this relaxed feeling yet, it will come during one of your next practice periods. The important thing is not to work hard on the exercises; try to do them as relaxed as possible. Your muscles are working even when you do the movements kind of sloppy. I know that is a terrible word to use as a phys. ed. teacher, but I found it is the best way to get people to do the exercises relaxed. When the muscles in your body are relaxed, also your mind, your nervous system and the organs in your body are relaxing. The blood can circulate easier because the tension is gone. After the relaxing period you feel beautifully refreshed and full of energy.

SUMMARY

FIRST WEEK'S EXERCISES.

WARM-UPS.

1. Arm Swinging.   10 X
2. Knee Raising.   10 X
3. Side Bend.   3 X each side.
4. Arm Circles.   10 X
5. Shoulders Rolling.   5 X
6. Squatting Down.   4 X
7. Stretching Up.   2 X

YOGA EXERCISES.

1. Balancing No. 1. Count to 10 on each foot.
2. Wide Knee Bend and Shift. 5 X each.
3. Triangle. 1 X to each side. Lie down and relax.
4. Hiprolls. 10 X in each direction.
5. Leg Raising. 2 X each leg. 2 X both legs.
6. Knee and Head Raising. 1 X each.
7. Both Knees Raising. 1 X
8. Neck Movements. 3 X each.
9. Rock and Roll. 8-10 X. Relax.
10. Half Shoulderstand. 2 X. Relax.
11. Bridge Posture. 3 X
12. Relaxing Posture. 10 minutes.

SECOND WEEK'S EXERCISES.

Today we are going to do the same exercises again we did in the first session because the constant repetition is a very important part of this systematic exercise routine. The muscles have to get used to these movements, the connective tissues have to be stretched so you can do the exercises every week more and more relaxed and gracefully.

But also some new exercises come into the routine or the old ones are changed slightly depending on the progress you are making. But *the sequence of the exercises always stays the same, because in each session the body has to be prepared step by step for the next exercise and the rules of the body mechanics are always the same.*

Today we start with the first Breathing Exercises which are a very important part of the Yoga Exercise system and also one of the most important parts for your well-being.

But first let's do the Warm-up exercises:
Sit up slowly over your right side and stand up slowly.

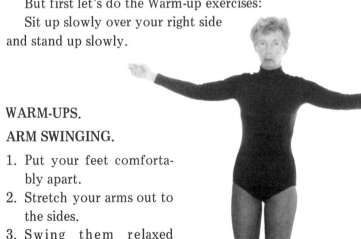

WARM-UPS.
ARM SWINGING.

1. Put your feet comfortably apart.
2. Stretch your arms out to the sides.
3. Swing them relaxed around your body.

10 X

2ND WEEK.

KNEE RAISING.

1. Put your feet together.
2. Raise your right knee up.
3. Put your right foot down.
   Repeat with your left leg.

      10 X count right knee.

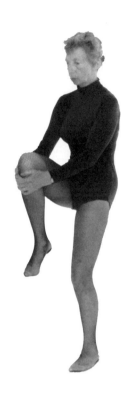

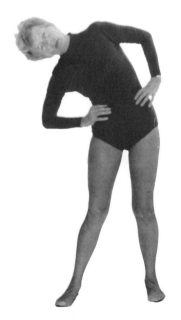

SIDE BEND.

1. Put your feet comfortably apart,
2. Your hands to your hips,
3. Bend your upper body gently to your right side,
4. And bend it to your left side.

      3 X to each side.

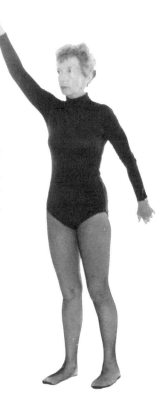

ARM CIRCLES.

1. Put your feet comfortably apart.
2. Stretch your right arm straight up.
3. Let it fall back and swing it around. Repeat with your left arm about 10 x each arm. If you can do it relaxed, try both arms: Stretch one arm forward, one back and swing them backwards simultaneously.

10 X

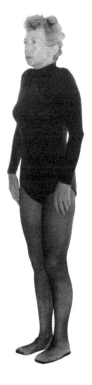

SHOULDER ROLLING.

1. Gently draw your shoulders up.
2. Then bring them back.
3. And down and around.

About 5 X

SQUATTING DOWN.

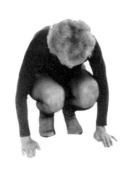

1. Put your feet slightly apart,
2. Bend your knees slowly,
3. Put your hands on the mat.
   Carry more weight on your hands than
   on your knees,
4. Come up slowly.

4 X

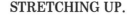

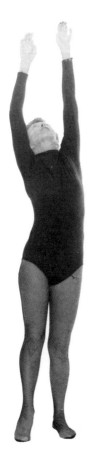

STRETCHING UP.

1. Put your feet comfortably apart.
2. Raise your arms over your head,
3. Stretch your right side up,
4. Stretch your left side up, 3 x each
   3 X each side.
5. Completely relaxed, bend your upper
   body down.
6. Come up slowly with your knees
   slightly bent.

2 X

These were the Warm-up exercises. Now the blood circulates well in every part of the body, the joints are limbered up, the muscles warmed up: we are ready for the slow motion Yoga exercises.

SECOND WEEK'S YOGA EXERCISES.

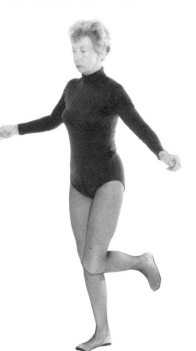

FIRST BALANCING EXERCISE.

1. Stand on your right foot.
2. Raise your arms slightly at your sides.
3. Lift your left foot up.
4. Put your knees together.
5. Concentrate on a spot 4-5 feet in front of you. Hold to the count of 10.
   Repeat on left foot.

If you practiced regularly during the week, you will feel that your muscles are stronger, you can stand more securely without wiggling. Now we can go on to the Second Balancing exercise. But if you cannot stand securely yet during the First Balancing exercise, then keep practicing it until you can stand on one foot relaxed and easily.

Some people who have problems balancing, can have insufficient blood circulation in the head, especially in the ears where the balancing system is located. If the problem lies here, it will get better through practicing the Half Shoulderstand, which increases the blood circulation in every organ of the head.

SECOND BALANCING EXERCISE.

1. Stand on your right foot.
2. Lift your left leg up slowly.
3. Reach for your toes with your left hand.
4. Stretch your right arm up, hold for a few seconds.
5. Bring arm and foot slowly down, relax your legs by shaking them slightly.

   Repeat on your left foot.

   Besides the balancing this gives the body a good stretch and prepares for more advanced balancing exercises.

   Caution: If pregnant, don't stretch too much, just raise arm.

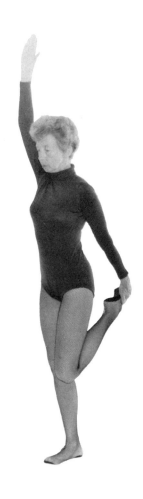

2ND WEEK.

WIDE KNEE BEND AND SHIFT.

1. Put your feet wider apart than is comfortable.
2. Keep feet parallel, toes pointing straight ahead.
3. Bend your right knee, keep left leg stretched.
4. Come up, shift over and bend your left knee.

5 X count right knee.

5. Now stay down and shift over from side to side, keep feet flat on mat.

8 X count right knee.

Every time you practice this exercise you will feel how your legs get stronger. If you are interested in losing around your upper legs, measure them now, write down what you measured and check it again in 3 months. But it only works if you do your exercises every day.

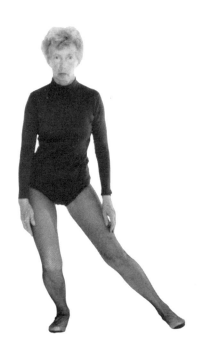

TRIANGLE POSTURE.

1. Put your feet comfortably apart.
2. Raise your arms palms up to shoulder height *during inhalation.*
3. Turn your right hand around, bend down to your right side, *exhale.*
4. Put your hand to the outside of your knee.
5. Bring your stretched left arm closer to your head until you feel a slight stretch along your side.
6. Slowly raise your body up, turn your hands around, *inhale.*
7. Bend down to your left side, *exhale.*
8. Put your hand to the outside of your knee.
9. Bring your stretched right arm closer to your head until you feel this gentle stretch again along your side.
10. Slowly raise your body up.

You will feel that you can stretch and reach a little bit farther every time you practice. The muscles and the connective tissues in your side are getting stretched gently. If it feels comfortable, then we start holding the posture for a few seconds. But you should never feel any strain, so start watching your body inside carefully.

From now on we do it with breathing.

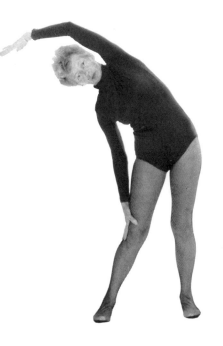

2ND WEEK.

HIPROLLS.

To relax the muscles we just stretched, let's do the Hiprolls.

1. Put your feet comfortably apart,
2. Your hands on your hips.
3. Roll your hips around gently.

10 X in each direction.

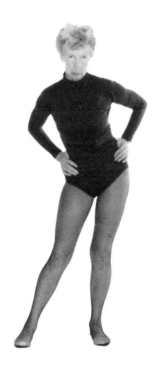

Lie down and relax.

THE FIRST BREATHING EXERCISES.

Today we start with the Breathing Exercises, which are an important part of the Yoga Exercise system, but the breathing is also the most important part of your life, your health and well being. Unfortunately most people have to learn how to breathe properly again. All small children breathe the normal, natural way, but when they get older, somebody tells them "keep your tummy in" and this results in breathing only with the upper part of their lungs. So most people and especially women who are wearing corsets and girdles, use only a small part of their lungs for breathing. Doctors are very concerned about the bad breathing habits of people today, because quite a number of ailments are the result of insufficient intake of oxygen into the lungs and consequently into the body and its cells.

The body also needs oxygen to utilize the food you eat. If you don't get enough oxygen into your body, the food cannot be assimilated and is stored on the spots where we don't need it and where it is so hard to get rid of it again. And you have this hungry feeling all the time. Breathe properly and you will utilize the food you are eating and you will be surprised how little food you really need.

To learn the normal, natural breathing again, we divide it into three parts:

1. The lower or abdominal breathing, also called diaphragmatic or belly breathing.
2. The middle or ribcage breathing.
3. The upper or chest breathing.

This normal natural breathing is done through the nose. We inhale and exhale through the nose. Only the nose has built in protection against dirt and dust. In the entrance of the nose are little hair screens which block dirt and dust from going farther back and into the lungs. There are long channels which warm up the cold air before it enters the lungs.

And in the nose we also have the device for scents and odors, the olfactory organ, which also absorbs with the oxygen the life energy of life force, which the Yogis call prana. This prana or this life force, that we take in with the oxygen stays in the body and gets stored so that whenever you need it in certain difficult times in your life, it will be there. But only through regular natural breathing, can you get enough of this prana into your body. You cannot get the prana into your body by breathing through the mouth. Whenever you have problems breathing through your nose, try to get your nose clear as soon as possible. Even a short time breathing through the mouth will get you tired and besides that, it is dangerous because there is no protection for your lungs. It is especially important to watch children; if they are breathing through the mouth, this habit should be changed to nose breathing. Otherwise it can result in retarded mental development and enlarged tonsils.

THE ABDOMINAL BREATHING. (Preparation.)

Now let's start with the first part of breathing, the abdominal breathing. For most people it is the hardest part to learn again. To make it easier, we start by just letting the tummy muscles relax and then contract them.

So lie on your back, bend your knees, feet on the mat. Put your hands on your tummy just below your belly button. Now let your tummy go out gently *(don't push it out)*, and draw it in slowly.

Just your tummy should move, nothing else, and don't think about breathing, just let your tummy move out and draw it in again. Slowly, relaxed, without any jerky movements.

Do that about 10 X.

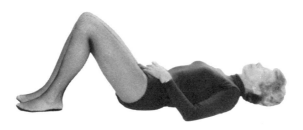

I know for most women it feels awful to let the tummy go out. But don't worry, you will not get a big tummy by doing this; on the contrary, through relaxing and contracting the muscles they will get stronger and you will get a nice firm tummy.

Now do the same exercise with your tummy muscles again and this time close your eyes and really watch what is going on in your body. You will feel when your tummy goes out, you are inhaling; when you draw your tummy in, you are exhaling. You cannot help it, it just works this way. This is the normal natural way to breathe. When you watch a small child breathe, you can see the gentle movement of the tummy. Also all animals breathe this way.

Now let's see what is going on inside of the body during the movements of your tummy muscles. When you let your tummy go out, your diaphragm can move down and your lungs can expand downwards. This creates a vacuum in the lowest part of your lungs and the fresh air or the oxygen goes all the way to the lowest part of your lungs. When you draw your tummy muscles in, they push against the diaphragm, that pushes against your lungs and pushes the stale air or the carbon dioxide out.

The lungs do not have muscles of their own, the breathing has to be done with the muscles around your lungs. These are on the bottom: The tummy muscles and the diaphragm (you cannot move the diaphragm at will, it only moves when you move your tummy muscles); in the middle breathing: The ribcage muscles; and in the upper breathing: The chest and shoulder muscles. When these muscles stretch or expand the lungs underneath can expand and can get filled with enough oxygen to supply every cell in your body. The more relaxed these muscles are the more they can expand and the more oxygen can get into your lungs.

Through the Yoga exercises we do, we relax all these muscles systematically and you will feel each day that the breathing will become easier and more and more relaxed.

THE ABDOMINAL BREATHING.

We learned the movement of the Abdominal Breathing and now we are going to do it while thinking about the breathing and really concentrating on it.

Lie there completely relaxed, bend your knees, feet on the mat. Put your hands on your tummy, direct your consciousness to your tummy.

All breathing exercises start with an exhalation to get the stale air out of your lungs.

1. So draw your tummy in and exhale through your nose,
2. Now let your tummy go out completely relaxed and inhale,
3. Draw your tummy in and exhale slowly and relaxed.

10 X

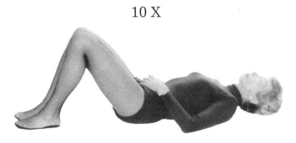

It is a very gentle and small movement and only your tummy should move, not your chest.

This abdominal breathing has a tremendous calming effect on your body, it relaxes your heart, your nervous system and your mind. If you have trouble falling asleep, do this gentle breathing. It also gives your abdominal organs a gentle massage and increases the peristaltic movements of your intestines, also increases the blood circulation in the abdominal organs to make them function properly.

The important thing is: *do not push your abdomen out.* Just let it go out easily and relaxed. It is a very small movement. If you would push it out, then you can get a big tummy. You can hardly see this movement, just feel it. That is the reason I let my students put the hands on the tummy so I can see this gentle movement.

THE MIDDLE OR RIBCAGE BREATHING.

1. Lie relaxed, put your hands on your ribcage. Direct your consciousness to your ribs.
2. Exhale through your nose, squeeze your ribs gently together, like pushing the air out.
3. Now expand your ribcage, during inhalation.
4. Feel your ribs moving together during exhalation.
   In the lying position you also feel your ribs raising but concentrate especially on the expansion. The more relaxed your muscles get, the easier you can expand your ribcage.

   Do it about 5 X. Don't work hard on it.

This ribcage breathing increases the blood circulation in your arms, hands and legs. If you have cold hands, you can immediately feel the tingling in your hands after doing the ribcage breathing.

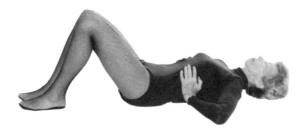

THE UPPER OR CHEST BREATHING.

1. Lie relaxed, put your fingertips on your collar bones.
2. Exhale through your nose, feel your chest going down.
3. Inhale slowly through raising your chest.
4. Exhale, feel your chest going down.

5 X

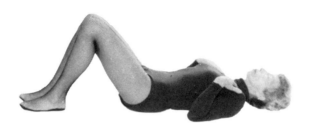

Most people can do this part easily because they breathe only this way. But if you breathe properly with this part, you should feel *the movement* of your chest; you will only get enough oxygen into your lungs when you really expand your chest and feel the oxygen entering your lungs.

These are the three parts of breathing. Please practice them every day. The best time to practice them is in the morning while you are still in bed. You are warm and relaxed and perhaps you have a few more minutes for yourself. Lie relaxed and do each part 5 X easily and relaxed. When you work with one part of breathing, don't worry about the other parts, just concentrate on one. And then try to practice the 3 parts of breathing again in the evening, just before you would like to go to sleep. Most of the time you will not get farther than the abdominal breathing before you fall asleep.

Next week we will put these three parts of breathing together to The Complete Breath.

Now lie there and relax.

53

LEG RAISING.

Strengthens back and abdominal muscles, firms up legs, hips, buttocks and tummy.

1. Lie on your back completely relaxed.
2. Raise your right leg slowly while inhaling.
3. Lower your right leg slowly while exhaling.
4. Raise your left leg slowly while inhaling.
5. Lower your left leg slowly while exhaling.

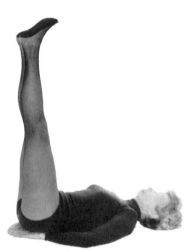

2 X

BOTH LEGS RAISING.

1. Put your hands under your buttocks, palms down.
2. Raise both legs slowly while inhaling.
3. Lower both legs slowly while exhaling. *Not if pregnant.*

2 X.

R e l a x.

It is important that the leg raising is done slowly, but again not too slowly, because then it could start straining the muscles. There is a certain slowness in the movements of the Yoga exercises. You will get the feeling after a few days of practice. Think about a slow motion picture sequence, how the movements flow slowly from the beginning to the end and you will get the right feeling for your movements.

2ND WEEK.

KNEE AND HEAD RAISING.

Relaxes the muscles in your lower back and stomach. Stretches and strengthens the upper back and neck muscles. Stretches the muscles in the upper leg.

1. Raise your arms over your head while inhaling — stretch and stretch.
2. Bring your right knee up to your chest, press it down — exhale.

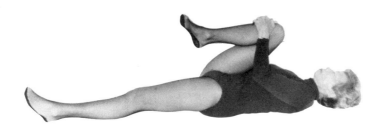

3. Gently raise your head toward your knee — inhale.
4. Put your head down — exhale.
5. Stretch your leg down, your arms up — inhale — stretch.
6. Bring your left knee up to your chest, press it down — exhale.
7. Gently raise your head toward your knee — inhale.
8. Put your head down — exhale.
9. Stretch your leg down, your arms up — inhale — stretch.
10. Bring your arms down — exhale and r e l a x.

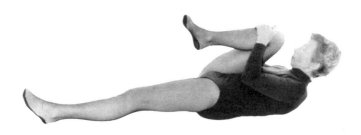

Close your eyes during this exercise and feel especially the beautiful stretch, then the relaxing effect when you raise the knee up, and the curling together when your head comes up too.

2ND WEEK.

RAISING BOTH KNEES.

Relaxes back and stomach muscles. Good position for a tired or strained back.

1. Raise your arms over your head while inhaling — s t r e t c h.
2. Bring both knees up to your chest, press them down — exhale.
3. Hold this position but relieve the pressure on your knees.
4. Breathe relaxed and consciously relax your back, relax your shoulders, relax your arms. Hold the position as long as you feel comfortable.
5. To come out of it, put your feet on the mat first, stretch your legs down, your arms up while inhaling — s t r e t c h.
6. Put your arms down — exhale and r e l a x.

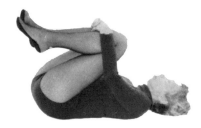

This should be a relaxing exercise. Do not raise your head when both knees are up. This would put too much strain on the neck muscles and could cause a headache. We only raise the head when one knee is up and we have the other outstretched leg as a counterbalance.

NECK RELAXING MOVEMENTS.

Relieves tension in the neck and upper back.

1. Sit in cross-legged position or on chair.
2. Slowly bring your head forward, chin toward chest.
3. Slowly raise your head up and let it go back as far as you can without any strain.

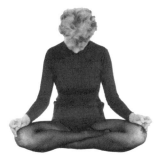
3 X
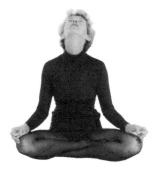

1. Turn your head to your right side slowly.
2. Slowly turn your head to your left side.

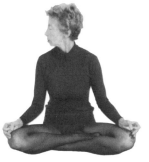
3 X
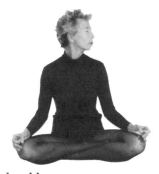

1. Tilt your head slowly toward your right shoulder.
2. Raise it up and tilt it slowly toward your left shoulder.

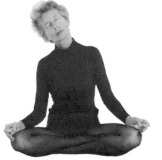
3 X
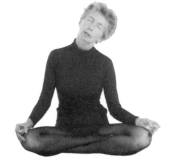

ROCK AND ROLL.

After relaxing your neck we now relax the back with the rock and roll exercise. Watch that your padding is thick enough. You should not feel the bones in your back when you roll.

1. Sit up, bend your knees, your feet on the mat.
2. Clasp your hands gently together under your knees.
3. Put your chin to your chest.
4. Swing your legs up gently and roll back to your shoulderblades.
5. Swing your legs down and roll up to feet on mat. Do it again and again relaxed and easy.

8-10 X

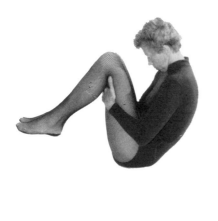
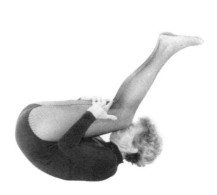

Lie down and relax.

You will feel more relaxed every time you practice the rock and roll. When you can roll up easily, then try to do it more slowly. Close your eyes and direct your consciousness to your spine, feel every vertebrae rolling down and up. But if you have trouble coming up, swing your legs down a little bit faster again.

THE HALF SHOULDERSTAND.

Increases the blood circulation in your neck and every part of the head.

1. Lying on your back put your hands under your buttocks, starting with palms down.
2. Slowly raise your legs and your hips, support them with your hands, elbows on the mat close to the body.
3. Hold this position for a few seconds. Legs in 45° angle.
4. To come down: First lower your legs slightly farther over your head.
5. Put your hands down on the mat, close together.
6. Bend your knees and slowly roll your back down, bring your hips down and bring your legs down.

Relax.

Repeat it after a few minutes of relaxing.

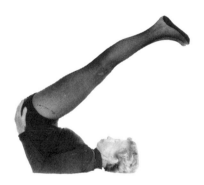

You will feel that it is easier to perform this exercise now than a week ago. If you still should have problems with raising your hips up, keep doing the "Leg Raising" exercise and the "Rock and Roll" until your muscles are strong enough to raise your hips up. Do not use a table or the wall to prop your legs up, you could easily strain a muscle. Your muscles will be able to do it on their own. Just be patient and keep practicing.

2ND WEEK.

BRIDGE POSTURE.

After the Half Shoulderstand we go into the Bridge Posture to bring the spine into the opposite movement from the Half Shoulderstand.

1. Lie on your back, arms relaxed alongside your body.
2. Bend your knees, put your feet on the mat close to your body about one foot apart.
3. Slowly raise your hips while inhaling.
4. Lower your hips while exhaling, press your back down, draw your tummy in.

3 X

Relax.

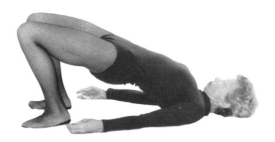

THE FORWARD BENDING EXERCISES.

The Forward Bending Exercises are the hardest exercises for most people. It will take a long time until you can reach your feet or put your forehead on your knee. *So take it easy and just reach to the point you can make easily.* You will get the benefits of this exercises in any case. It stretches the muscles and the connective tissues in the back of your legs (the hamstrings) and in your lower back. It is not your spine which is not flexible, it is the tightness of the connective tissue which prevents you from going down further. Through gently stretching it regularly, you will be able to bend down a little bit more every week. The exercise also increases the blood circulation in your abdominal organs and helps to reduce your tummy.

1. Sit on the floor and spread your legs apart.
2. Slowly raise your arms at your sides over your head while inhaling (to expand the ribcage).
3. Put your hands on your right knee or leg and bend down while exhaling.
4. Slide your hands up your leg, raise your arms at your sides over your head — inhale.
5. Bend down over your left leg while exhaling.

2 X

1. Bring your legs together, raise your arms while inhaling.
2. Bend down over both legs while exhaling.

2 X

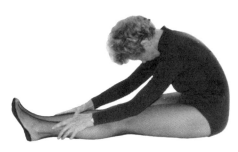

Relax your legs by gently shaking them.

THE ALTERNATE LEG BEND.

Combines the benefits of the Forward Bend with a gentle stretch of the knee tendons and muscles.

1. In the sitting position spread your legs apart.
2. Bend your left knee and put the sole against the inside of your right thigh.
3. Raise your arms at your sides over your head while inhaling.
4. Bend slowly over your right stretched leg while exhaling.
2 X

5. Stretch your leg, then bend your right knee and put the sole against the inside of your left thigh.
6. Raise your arms at your sides over your head while inhaling.
7. Bend slowly over your stretched leg while exhaling.
2 X

8. Stretch your leg, relax your legs by gently shaking them. Lie down and relax.

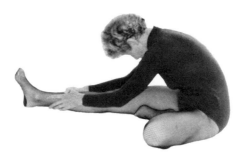

2ND WEEK.

THE PLANE.

After the Forward Bending Exercises we will stretch the whole body. This exercise also works on strengthening the wrists, upper arms, shoulders and upper back. It firms up the upper arms.

1. In the sitting position put your hands behind you in the most comfortable way.
2. Slowly raise your hips while inhaling, stretch your whole body, let your head go back.
3. Lower your hips while exhaling.

2 X

Do not stretch your feet down, just keep them relaxed. They will come down by themselves after a few weeks of practice when you will be able to raise your hips higher up. Forcing your feet down can cause cramps.

After the exercise, relax your wrists, relax your arms, relax your legs by gently shaking them.

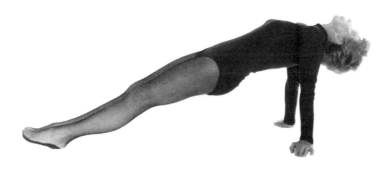

Lie down and relax.

2ND WEEK.

THE RELAXING POSTURE.

Close your eyes and lie in the most comfortable position. Slide your arms a few inches away from your body and turn your hands palms up. When you do this the first time it does not feel as relaxed as it should, but after a few times it will relax your shoulders and upper back muscles better and you will feel very comfortable this way.

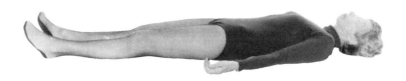

Relax your legs,
Relax your feet,
Relax your toes,
Relax your calves,
Relax your thighs,
Relax your stomach,
Relax your chest,
Relax your shoulders,
Relax your arms,
Relax your hands,
Relax your fingers,
Relax your neck,
Relax your head,
Relax your face,
Relax your mouth,
Relax your teeth,
Relax every muscle in your back,
Relax your whole body.

Relax for about 10-15 minutes, then raise your arms over your head and s t r e t c h, roll on your left side and s t r e t c h, roll on your right side and s t r e t c h, sit up over your right side.

2ND WEEK.

SECOND WEEK'S EXERCISES.

WARM-UPS.

1. Arm Swinging.   10 X
2. Knee Raising.   10 X
3. Side Bend.   3 X each side.
4. Arm Circles.   10 X both arms.
5. Shoulders Rolling   5 X
6. Squatting Down.   4 X
7. Stretching Up.   2 X

YOGA EXERCISES.
1. First Balancing exercise. To count of 10 each foot.
2. *Second Balancing Exercise.* To count of 5 each foot.
3. Wide Knee Bend and Shift. 8 X each.
4. Triangle. 1 X to each side.
5. Hiprolls. 10 X in each direction. Lie down and relax.
6. *Abdominal Breathing.* 10 X
7. *Middle or Ribcage Breathing.* 5 X
8. *Upper or Chest Breathing.* 5 X
9. Leg Raising. 2 X each.
10. Knee and Head Raising. 1 X each. Relax.
11. Neck Movements. 3 X each.
12. Rock and Roll. 8-10 X. Relax.
13. Half Shoulderstand. 2 X. Relax.
14. Bridge. 3 X. Relax.
15. *Forward Bend.* 2 X each.
16. *Alternate Leg Bend.* 2 X each side. Relax.
17. *The Plane.* 2 X
18. Relaxing Posture.

2ND WEEK.

The new exercises of this week are underlined. Do them gently, feel your way into them. If you think they are not yet comfortable to do, then keep practicing the others, but try them after a few days again. It is amazing how fast your body gets more flexible if you keep practicing regularly in this sequence.

THIRD WEEK'S EXERCISES.

Now after two weeks of practicing the Yoga exercises you are not a straight beginner any more. You already feel your body, you know it better and can watch it well. And I hope you feel better all over. Today we add a few more exercises, which work on muscles you have not used for a long time. This is the amazing thing about the Yoga exercise system, it works with every muscle and every part in your body to bring them to good working order and good condition.

So first lie down and relax for a few minutes and get into the mood for your exercises.

Then sit up slowly over your right side, stand up slowly and let's start with the Warm-Up Exercises.

By now you should know them by heart and I just write the titles and the number of how often to do them.

WARM-UPS.

1. Arm Swinging.	10 X
2. Knee Raising.	10 X
3. Side Bend.	3 X
4. Arm Circles. If you can do it relaxed, then do both arms simultaneously backwards.	10 X
5. Shoulders Rolling.	5 X
6. Squatting Down.	4 X
7. Stretching Up.	2 X

THIRD WEEK'S YOGA EXERCISES.

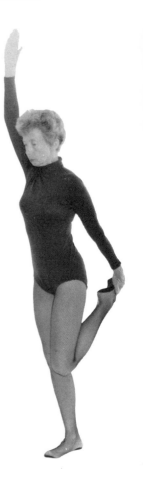

SECOND BALANCING EXCERCISE.

1. Stand on your right foot.
2. Lift your left leg up slowly.
3. Reach for your toes with your left hand.
4. Stretch your right arm up.
5. Hold to the count of 10.
6. Bring arm and foot down slowly. Repeat on your left foot.

   Relax your legs by gently shaking them.

If you have problems with this balancing exercise, then stand close to the wall, lift the outside foot up hold on with your hand. With hand close to the wall crawl up the wall until your arm is stretched out, then let go. Just the feeling of having the wall nearby makes it easier to balance. After a few times you will be able to do it without the wall.

3RD WEEK.

WIDE KNEE BEND AND SHIFT.

1. Put your feet wider apart than is comfortable.
2. Keep feet parallel, toes pointing straight ahead.
3. Bend your right knee, keep left leg stretched.
4. Come up, shift over and bend left knee.

10 X count right knee.

1. Now stay down and shift from side to side.

10 X count right knee.

If you feel your legs are getting stronger, go down a bit deeper every time you practice.

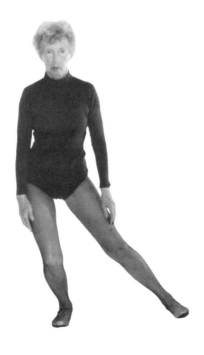

TRIANGLE POSTURE.

1. Put your feet comfortably apart.
2. Raise your arms, palms up, to shoulder height while inhaling.
3. Turn your right hand around, bend down to your right side — exhale.
   Hold the position about 5 seconds, do a gentle abdominal breathing.
4. Slowly raise your body up, turn your hands around — inhale.
5. Bend down to your left side — exhale.
   Hold the position about 5 seconds, do a gentle abdominal breathing.
6. Slowly raise your body up.

We will now start to hold the position a few seconds. But watch your body carefully. You should not feel any strain, just a gentle stretch. If you feel a strain, then do not hold it yet. Your muscles need some more time to get limber, so do not force anything.

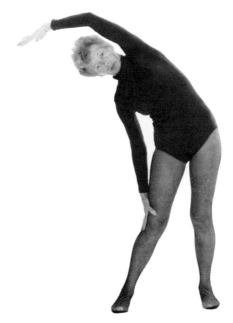

70

3RD WEEK.

HIPROLLS.

Especially when we start to hold the Triangle Posture for a few seconds, you will feel how good the Hiprolls are to relax the muscles we just stretched.

1. Put your feet comfortably apart.
2. Your hands on your hips.
3. Roll your hips around gently.

10 X in each direction.

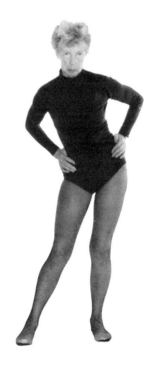

Lie down and relax.

3RD WEEK.

THE BREATHING EXERCISES.

Today we start to do the breathing exercises in the sitting position. We can do them sitting cross-legged or if you feel more comfortable, sit on a chair, but in any case try to sit straight to make the breathing easier.

THE ABDOMINAL BREATHING.

1. Sit cross-legged or on a chair, put your hands on your tummy. Close your eyes and concentrate on your breath.
2. Draw your tummy in — exhale.
3. Let your tummy go out — inhale.
4. Draw your tummy in — exhale.

10 X slowly and relaxed.

Only your tummy should move.

Stretch your legs, relax your legs by shaking them gently.

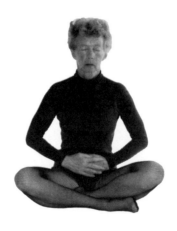

THE MIDDLE OR RIBCAGE BREATHING.

1. Sit cross-legged or on a chair.
2. Put your hands on your ribcage.
3. Squeeze your ribs gently together — exhale.
4. Expand your ribcage — inhale.
5. Feel your ribs moving together — exhale.

5 X slowly and relaxed.

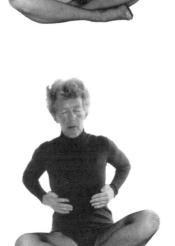

Stretch your legs, relax your legs by shaking them gently.

The ribcage breathing feels different in the sitting position than in the lying position. Now you feel only the expansion; when you are lying down, you also feel a raising movement, because the muscles in the back are restricted in their movement.

When you do the ribcage breathing the first few times in the sitting position, you will not feel too much expansion of your ribcage, because these muscles are very tight. Only if you like to sing or you swim regularly, do you know how to expand your ribcage. But most people have to learn it. These muscles cannot be moved easily like you would move your hands or arms. You really have to concentrate on it. I found the easiest way to practice the ribcage breathing is:

Stand in front of the mirror, put your hands on your ribs — exhale — and squeeze your ribs gently together. Put your fingertips together. Then look in the mirror and inhale by expanding your ribcage and you can see how your fingertips move apart; in the beginning just perhaps half an inch, later on, two to three inches. Let your ribs move together and exhale. There should be only an expansion not a raising of the ribcage or the chest.

3RD WEEK.

THE UPPER OR CHEST BREATHING.

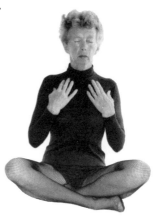

1. Sit cross-legged or on a chair.
2. Put your hands on your collar bones.
3. Exhale through your nose, feel your chest going down.
4. Inhale slowly through raising your chest, expanding your shoulders.
5. Exhale — feel your chest going down.

5 X

Stretch your legs, relax your legs by shaking them gently.

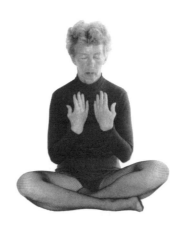

FOOT EXERCISES.

Before we go on to the next breathing exercise, we will relax the legs and feet and do some stretching and limbering up with your feet and ankles. These movements will make your ankles more flexible and we need flexible ankles for quite a number of Yoga exercises. They also will increase the blood circulation in your feet and legs and will slim down and firm up your legs and ankles.

1. In the sitting position, put your hands behind you.
2. Stretch your feet, but don't point your toes, stretch your instep.
3. Stretch your heels, feel a gentle stretch in back of your calves.

5 X

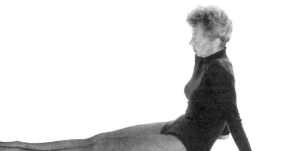

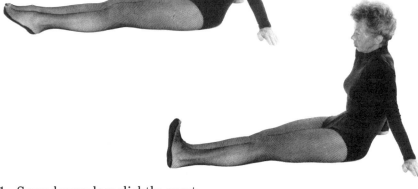

1. Spread your legs slightly apart.
2. Roll your feet around in gentle circles.
3. Roll them in the opposite directions slowly and relaxed.

5 X in each direction

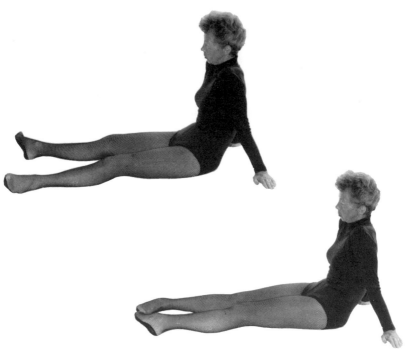

1. Raise your right leg slightly and shake it, put it down.
2. Raise your left leg slightly and shake it, put it down.
3. Raise both legs slightly and shake them, put them down. Relax your legs.

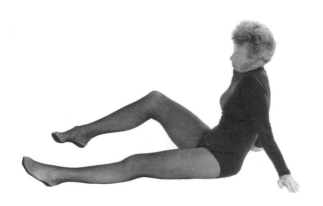

THE COMPLETE BREATH.

Now let's put the 3 parts of Breathing together to one complete breath.

1. Sit cross-legged or on a chair. Put your hands on your tummy, close your eyes, concentrate on your breath.
2. Draw your tummy in and exhale through your nose.
3. Let your tummy go out relaxed while inhaling through your nose, expand your ribcage and raise your chest.
4. Draw your tummy in while exhaling, your ribs move together, the chest goes down.

3 X

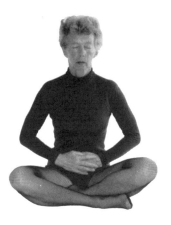

Lie down and relax.

It is a wavelike motion through your body. When you start filling the middle part of your lungs, you will feel that your tummy already goes in by itself. Don't fight that; this is the natural way of breathing. But when you exhale, draw your tummy in a little bit tighter. Then your ribs go together and your chest goes down. You will also notice that you don't have to inhale right away again, because after a deep breath like that you take a short rest and automatically your body will inhale again. The breathing always starts with the lowest part of your lungs, the inhalation starts with the abdominal breathing and the exhalation also starts with the lowest part of your lungs. The air goes out in the same sequence in which it was admitted.

The first few times practicing the complete breath, you will have some difficulties. Just do it as relaxed as possible. Don't work hard on it. It is the natural breathing and in a short time your body will learn it. With each breath you should fill your whole lungs with oxygen, so the millions of tiny air sacs in your lungs can bring the oxygen into your bloodstream, the bloodstream bringing it to all the cells in your body. Every cell in your body needs the oxygen to function properly. If you do not bring oxygen into every part of your lungs with every breath, quite a large number of cells in your body do not get the oxygen they need and start suffering. These are the spots where the trouble starts.

Breathe with the complete breath and you will feel better, more alive, full of energy and you will not tire so easily.

The Complete Breath also calms your nervous system and gives you a beautiful relaxed feeling.

Practice The Three Parts of Breathing and The Complete Breath every morning and every evening in bed, when you are relaxed. Really concentrate on it and feel the oxygen coming into your body and feel the stale air or the carbon dioxide moving out. And always remember this breathing is done only through your nose. We only have some special breathing exercises, where we exhale through the mouth to accomplish a special effect.

THE LEG RAISING.

1. Lie completely relaxed, arms alongside your body.
2. Raise your right leg slowly while inhaling.
3. Lower your right leg slowly while exhaling.
4. Raise your left leg while inhaling.
5. Lower your left leg while exhaling.

2 X

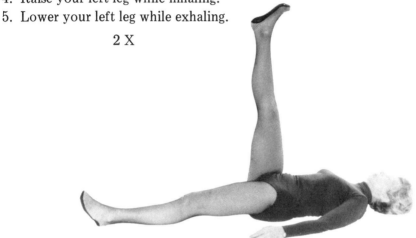

1. Put your hands under your buttocks, palms down.
2. Raise both legs slowly while inhaling.
3. Lower both legs while exhaling.

   Should not be done if pregnant.

2 X

Relax.

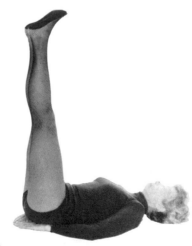

KNEE AND HEAD RAISING.

1. Raise your arms over your head while inhaling — s t r e t c h.
2. Bring your right knee up to your chest, press it down — exhale.
3. Gently raise your head toward your knee — inhale.
4. Put your head down — exhale (feel the neck muscles relax).
5. Stretch your leg down, your arms up — inhale — s t r e t c h.
6. Bring your left knee up to your chest, press it down — exhale.
7. Gently raise your head toward your knee — inhale.
8. Put your head down — exhale.
9. Stretch your leg down, your arms up — inhale — s t r e t c h.
10. Bring your arms down — exhale and relax.

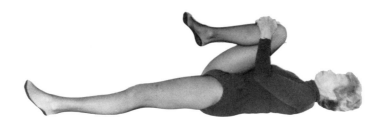

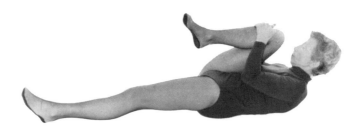

BOTH KNEES RAISING.

1. Raise your arms over your head while inhaling — s t r e t c h.
2. Bring both knees up to your chest, press them down — exhale.
3. Hold this position but relieve the pressure on your knees.
4. Breathe relaxed and consciously relax your back,
   relax your shoulders,
   relax your arms.
5. Then put your feet on the mat first, stretch your legs down, your arms up, while inhaling — s t r e t c h.
6. Put your arms down — exhale and r e l a x.

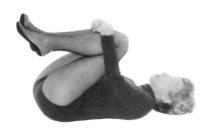

NECK RELAXING MOVEMENTS.

1. Sit in cross-legged position or on chair.
2. Slowly bring your head down, chin to chest.
3. Slowly raise your head up and bring it back.

5 X

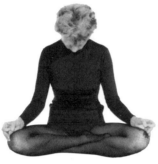 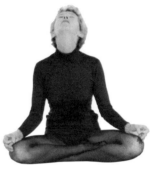

1. Turn your head slowly to your right side.
2. Turn your head slowly to your left side.

5 X

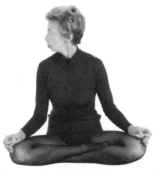 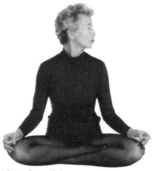

1. Tilt your head slowly toward your right shoulder.
2. Raise it up and tilt it slowly toward your left shoulder.

5 X

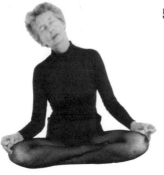 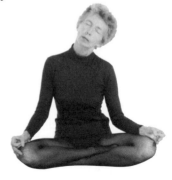

ROCK AND ROLL.

1. Sit up, bend your knees, feet on the mat.
2. Clasp your hands gently together under your knees.
3. Put your chin to your chest.
4. Swing your legs up gently and roll back to your shoulderblades.
5. Swing your legs down and roll up.

8-10 X

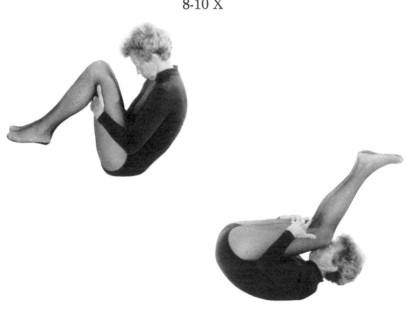

Lie down and r e l a x.

THE HALF SHOULDERSTAND.

1. Lie on your back, put your hands under your buttocks, starting with palms down.
2. Slowly raise your legs and hips, support them with your hands.
3. Hold this position for 10 seconds. Do a gentle abdominal breathing.
4. To come down: Lower your legs slightly farther over your head.
5. Put your hands down on the mat, close together.
6. Bend your knees and slowly roll your back down, bring your hips down, they should come automatically on your hands and stretch your legs down. R e l a x.

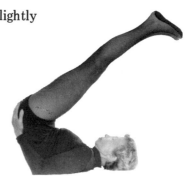

2 X

Only hold the position if you can do it easily and relaxed without feeling any strain in your back.

BRIDGE POSTURE.

1. Lie on your back, arms relaxed alongside your body.
2. Bend your knees, put your feet on the mat about one foot apart.
3. Slowly raise your hips while inhaling.
4. Lower your hips while exhaling, press your back down, draw your tummy in.

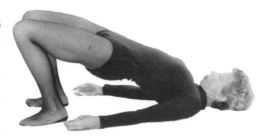

3 X

R e l a x.

84

3RD WEEK.

FORWARD BEND.

1. Sit up and spread your legs apart.
2. Slowly raise your arms at your sides over your head while inhaling.
3. Put your hand on your right knee or leg, bend down while exhaling.
4. Slide your hands up your leg, raise your arms at your sides over your head while inhaling.
5. Bend down over your left leg while exhaling.

2 X

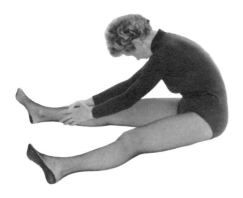

1. Put your legs together, raise your arms while inhaling.
2. Bend down over both legs while exhaling.

2 X

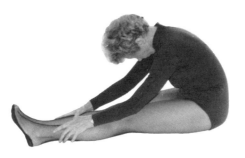

Relax your legs by shaking them gently.

THE ALTERNATE LEG BEND.

1. In the sitting position spread your legs apart.
2. Put the sole of your left foot against the inside of your right thigh.
3. Raise your arms at your sides over your head while inhaling.
4. Bend slowly over your stretched leg while exhaling.

2 X

Stretch your leg, relax your legs.

1. Spread your legs apart again.
2. Put the sole of your right foot against the inside of your left thigh.
3. Raise your arms at your sides over your head while inhaling.
4. Bend slowly over your stretched leg while exhaling.

2 X

Stretch your leg, relax your legs.

Lie down and relax.

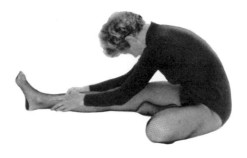

3RD WEEK.

THE PLANE.

Now let's stretch the whole body.

1. In the sitting position put your hands behind you in the most comfortable way.
2. Slowly raise your hips while inhaling, stretch your whole body, let your head go back.
3. Lower your hips slowly while exhaling.

2 X

Relax your wrists, relax your arms, relax your legs by gently shaking them.

Lie down and relax.

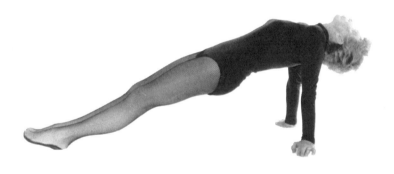

3RD WEEK.

SPINAL TWIST. (First version.)

With the preceding exercises we did bend the spine in different directions. Now we give the spine a gentle twist. It stretches the muscles in the sides and the diagonal muscles of the back and neck. It is a movement we seldom do, so we have to do it very carefully.

1. Sit up straight, keep your right leg stretched out.
2. Put your left foot over your right knee, parallel to your leg.
3. Put your right hand on your left foot.
4. Stretch your left arm forward, keep looking at your hand and slowly bring your left arm back as far as you can without feeling any strain.
5. Bring your arm slowly forward, looking at your hand.
6. Put your arm down, stretch your leg, relax your legs.

Now the other side.

1. Sit up straight, keep your left leg stretched out.
2. Put your right foot over your left knee, parallel to your leg.
3. Put your left hand on your right foot.
4. Stretch your right arm forward, keep looking at your right hand and slowly bring your right arm back as far as you can without feeling any strain.
5. Bring your arm slowly forward again, looking at your hand.
6. Put your arm down, stretch your leg, relax your legs.

Lie down and relax.

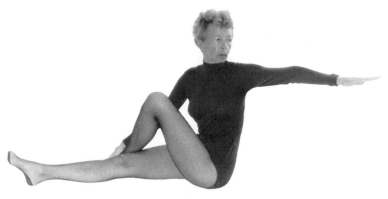

BACK EXERCISES. (a)

To stretch and to limber up the muscles in the back. These next movements should be done especially gently and carefully, because the back and the neck muscles are the stiffest and tightest muscles in most people. If you have a swayback put a towel, folded together, under your tummy.

1. Lie on your stomach and stretch your arms forward.
2. Slowly raise your right arm and your head while inhaling, keep stretching forward. Don't raise too high, about 5-10 inches.
3. Put your arm and head down — exhale.
4. Raise your left arm and your head while inhaling.
5. Put your arm and head down — exhale.

2 X

If you have trouble raising your head, don't try too hard. Just wait a few more weeks for it. All the other exercises we will do will strengthen and relax your neck muscles and in a few more weeks you will be able to do it.

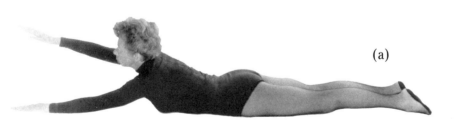

(a)

BACK EXERCISE. (b)

To strengthen and to stretch the muscles in the lower back.

1. Lie on your stomach, hands under your chin.
2. Slowly raise your right leg while inhaling — keep feet relaxed.
3. Lower your leg — exhale.
4. Raise your left leg while inhaling.
5. Lower your leg while exhaling.

2 X

Close your eyes and watch the muscles in your lower back. You should not feel any strain, just a gentle stretch. Keep your feet relaxed.

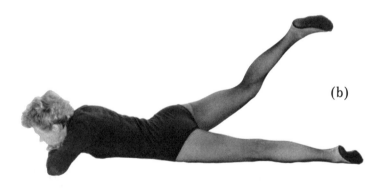

(b)

BACK EXERCISE. No. 1.

Now we put these last two exercises together into one exercise. Do it very carefully and watch your body inside. Be aware of what is going on and of how your muscles work. *Do not do this exercise if pregnant.*

1. Lie on your stomach, stretch your arms forward.
2. Keep stretching forward, slowly raise your right arm, your left leg and head while inhaling.
3. Lower arm, leg and head while exhaling.
4. Slowly raise your left arm, your right leg and your head while inhaling.
5. Lower your arm, leg and head while exhaling.

2 X

Even if you don't like these last three exercises too much in the beginning, keep practicing them. They are preparing your body for more advanced exercises and are also absolutely necessary to limber up and to stretch the long muscles in your back, helping to prevent back problems.

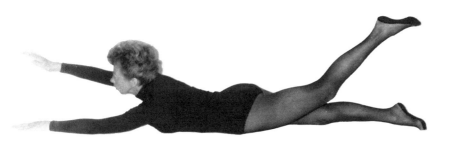

No. 1

3RD WEEK.

THE PUSH-UP.

To strengthen wrists and upper arms, also to firm up upper arms, which easily get flabby, if they are not used often enough.

1. Lie on your stomach, put your hands under your shoulders.
2. Bend your knees or just keep your knees on the floor.
3. Push your upper body up during inhalation — slowly.
4. Lower your body during exhalation — slowly.

5 X

Lie down and relax.

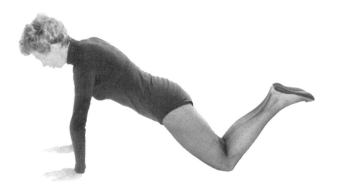

This is the modified way of doing push-ups. We would like to strengthen wrists and arms. Men have stronger wrists and arms from the beginning and can do the push-up from the toes without having the knees resting on the mat. In both cases it is important to keep the body straight, so the weight is carried by the arms and not by the legs. Women should not be afraid to do push-ups; it does not develop big arm muscles, just strengthens them, making the exercises which follow in the next few weeks easier.

WORKING UP TO PUSH-UPS.

If you have trouble doing the modified push-ups, it may be because of wrist problems (broken wrist, sprained wrist) or overweight. Here is a way to work slowly up to them, and strengthen the wrists and arms gradually. With this exercise you also stretch your hamstring muscles. (Good for joggers and runners.)

1. Stand in front of the wall facing it, about one foot away.
2. Put your hands against the wall, fingers pointing to each other.
3. With resistance bring your forehead to the wall.
4. With resistance push your body away from it.

5 X

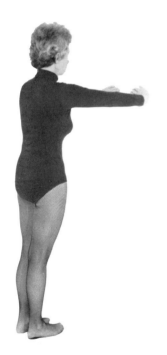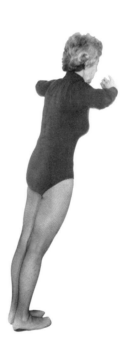

You can put as much strength into it as you want to do. Try to increase it every day. It is important that you keep the body in one straight line. After a week of practice step a few inches farther back. Keep heels down.

YOGA MUDRA. (SYMBOL OF YOGA.)

A beautiful relaxing position for the muscles in the back and for every organ in your body. All activity in your body is slowed down. In the beginning it is not a very relaxing position for everybody. But after a short time when your ankles are flexible enough so you can easily sit back on your heels, it will become a very comfortable pose.

1. Sit back on your heels.
2. Raise your arms sideways over your head while inhaling.
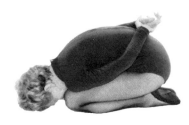
3. Bend forward slowly while exhaling, keep sitting on your heels, put your hands behind your back, hold your right wrist.
4. Put your head (forehead or top) on the floor.
5. Hold the position and do a gentle abdominal breathing.
   Hold to the count of 10.
6. Slowly raise your body up. Go on your hands and knees, put your feet over to one side, your hand down on the other side, sit down beside your hand, stretch your legs, relax your legs, lie down and r e l a x. (Lying down this way from sitting on your heels avoids straining your knee cartilage.

If you should feel a slight pressure in your head or neck during the Yoga Mudra pose, put your fists on top of each other in front of you and put your head on the top fist. Your body is still in the relaxing position, but your head is not in the inverted position. People with high blood pressure should always do it with their fists in front.

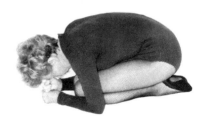

3RD WEEK.

THE RELAXING POSTURE.

Lie down and relax in the most comfortable position. Close your eyes and concentrate on the parts of your body I am going to mention.

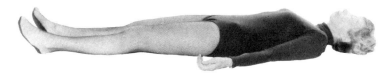

Relax your legs,
Relax your feet,
Relax your toes,
Relax your calves,
Relax your thighs,
Relax your stomach,
Relax your chest,
Relax your shoulders,
Relax your arms,
Relax your hands,
Relax your fingers,
Relax your neck,
Relax your head,
Relax four face,
Relax your mouth,
Relax your teeth,
Relax every muscle in your back,
Relax your whole body.
Relax completely.

If you should not feel relaxed enough yet, go through every part of your body again until you really feel relaxed.

After about 10 minutes raise your arms over your head and stretch your whole body, then roll on your left side and stretch, roll on your right side and stretch, and sit up over your right side.

Now we did all the exercises which are on the record: "Yoga For Beginners."* To get the right timing for your exercises, it would be beneficial, if you could practice with the record a few times.

---

*To obtain the record, find out if your local Health Food Store carries them. If not write to:
Ruth Bender
P. O. Box 414
Avon, Connecticut 06001
and ask for an order form.

3RD WEEK.

SUMMARY

THIRD WEEK'S EXERCISES.

WARM-UPS.

1. Arm Swinging.   10 X
2. Knee Raising.   10 X
3. Side Bend.   3 X each side.
4. Arm Circles.   10 X
5. Shoulders Rolling.   5 X
6. Squatting Down.   4 X
7. Stretching Up.   2 X

YOGA EXERCISES.

1. Second Balancing Exercise. Hold to count of 10 each foot.
2. Wide Knee Bend and Shift. 10 X
3. Triangle Posture. Hold 5 seconds.
4. Hiprolls. 10 X each direction.
5. *The Three Parts of Breathing. Sitting.*
   The Abdominal Breathing. 10 X
   The Middle Breathing. 5 X
   Upper Breathing. 5 X
6. *Foot Exercises.* 5 X each.
7. *The Complete Breath.* 3 X
8. The Leg Raising. 2 X each.
9. Knee and Head Raising. 1 X each.
10. Neck Relaxing Movement. 5 X each.
11. Rock and Roll. 8-10 X. Relax.
12. Half Shoulderstand. Hold 10 seconds. Relax.
13. Bridge Posture. 3 X. Relax.
14. Forward Bend. 2 X each.
15. The Alternate Leg Bend. 2 each.
16. The Plane. 2 X. Relax.
17. *Spinal Twist. 1st Version.* 1 X each side. Relax.

97

3RD WEEK.

18. *Back Exercises. a, b, No. 1.* 2 X each.
19. *The Push-Up.* 5 X
    Alternate Push-Ups (Wall).
20. *Yoga Mudra.* 1 X
21. Relaxing Posture.

98

4TH WEEK.

FOURTH WEEK'S EXERCISES.

During last week's exercise session you noticed that we started holding some of the exercises for a few seconds. In the beginning I call the movements exercises. When we start holding them they are called postures or in sanskrit "asanas." To hold the postures is the final goal we are working for. As a beginner it is hard to hold the postures, because the muscles are not strong, flexible and relaxed enough to endure it. But step by step you will be able to do it easier and relaxed. The longer you can hold the postures relaxed, the greater are the benefits you get out of it. But do not hurry anything; always watch your body. You will also feel that on some days you can hold a position more easily than on other days. The body is not in the same condition every day. Also the time of the day plays a role, so always be aware of the state your body is in. Then you get the results of the postures you would like to get.

So lie down and relax and feel your body. Just think about yourself only for a change and don't worry about anything else. Only if your body is in good condition and good health can you fulfill perfectly what you choose to do in your life.

Now sit up slowly over your right side.

Stand up slowly and let's start with the Warm-Up Exercises.

4TH WEEK.

WARM-UP EXERCISES.

      1. Arm Swinging.   10 X

      2. Knee Raising.   10 X

      3. Side Bend.   3 X

      4. Arm Circles.   10 X

      5. Shoulders Rolling.   5 X

      6. Squatting Down.   4 X

      7. Stretching Up.   2 X

FOURTH WEEK'S YOGA EXERCISES.

SECOND BALANCING EXERCISE.

1. Stand on your right foot.
2. Lift your left leg up slowly.
3. Reach for your toes with your left hand.
4. Stretch your right arm up.
5. Hold to the count of 10.
6. Bring arm and foot down slowly.
   Repeat on your left foot.

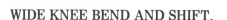

WIDE KNEE BEND AND SHIFT.

1. Put your feet wider apart than comfortable.
2. Keep your feet parallel, toes pointing straight ahead.
3. Bend your right knee, keep left leg stretched.
4. Come up, shift over and bend left knee.

   10 X, count right knee.

1. Stay down and shift from side to side.

   10 X, count right knee.

101

TRIANGLE POSTURE.

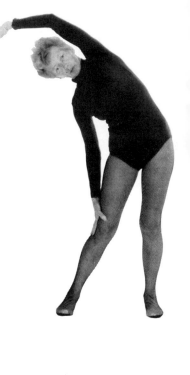

1. Put your feet comfortably apart.
2. Raise your arms, palms up to shoulder height while inhaling.
3. Turn your right hand around, bend down to your right side — exhale. Hold the position about 5 seconds with a gentle abdominal breathing.
4. Slowly raise your body up, turn your hands around — inhale.
5. Bend down to your left side — exhale.
   Hold 5 seconds. Do a gentle abdominal breathing.
6. Slowly raise your body up.

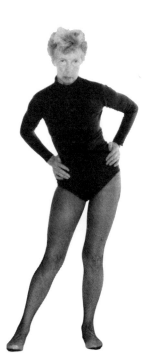

HIPROLLS.

1. Put your feet comfortably apart.
2. Your hands on your hips.
3. Roll your hips gently around.

   10 X in each direction.

PREPARATION FOR THE SUN EXERCISE.

UPPER LEG STRETCH.

1. Kneel down, put your hands in front of you.
2. Put your right foot forward between your hands.
3. Put your whole weight on your right foot, bring your knee forward. Feel the beautiful stretch in your leg.
4. Stretch your left leg back, resting on the knee.
5. Put your fingertips down beside your right foot.
6. Raise your head gently — inhale.
7. Put your head down exhale.
8. Bring your right knee back to your left knee, relax your legs.

Repeat with your left leg.

Stretches the muscles in your upper leg, slims down and firms up. Makes your ankles and knee joints more flexible. If you cannot touch your fingertips on the mat in the beginning, don't worry about it. When you muscles get stretched more and your ankles get more flexible you will be able to do it.

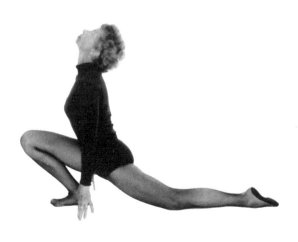

4TH WEEK.

PREPARATION FOR THE SUN EXERCISE.

HAMSTRING STRETCH.

1. Kneel down, put your hands in front of you.
2. Curl in your toes and stretch your legs.
3. Keep your feet and hands where they are.
4. *Gently and carefully* bring your heels down a little bit. *Don't Bounce,* go only as far as you can without feeling any strain.
5. Kneel down and relax your legs.

Repeat once.

Relax your legs.

From the kneeling position put your feet over to one side, sit down on the other side. Stretch your legs, relax your legs, lie down and relax.

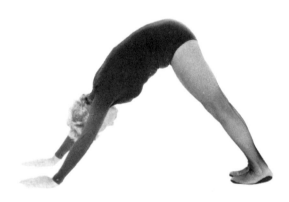

THE BREATHING EXERCISES.

THE ABDOMINAL BREATHING.

1. Sit cross-legged or on a chair, put your hands on your tummy.
2. Draw your tummy in — exhale.
3. Let your tummy go out completely relaxed — inhale.
4. Draw your tummy in — exhale.

5 X

Stretch your legs, relax your legs by gently shaking them.

THE MIDDLE OR RIBCAGE BREATHING.

1. Sit cross-legged or on a chair.
2. Put your hands on your ribcage.
3. Squeeze your ribs gently together — exhale.
4. Expand your ribcage — inhale.
5. Feel your ribs moving together — exhale.

5 X

Stretch your legs, relax your legs by gently shaking them.

THE UPPER OR CHEST BREATHING.

1. Sit cross-legged or on a chair.
2. Put your fingertips on your collarbones.
3. Exhale through your nose, feel your chest go down.
4. Inhale slowly by raising your chest, expanding your shoulders.
5. Exhale, feel your chest going down.

5 X

Stretch your legs, relax your legs by gently shaking them.

4TH WEEK.

FOOT EXERCISES.

1. In the sitting position put your hands behind you.
2. Stretch your feet, but don't point your toes, stretch your instep.
3. Stretch your heels, feel a gentle stretch in back of your calves.

5 X

1. Spread your legs slightly apart.
2. Roll your feet around in gentle circles.
3. Roll them in the opposite directions slowly and relaxed.

5 X

1. Raise your right leg slightly and shake it — put it down.
2. Raise your left leg slightly and shake it — put it down.
3. Raise both legs slightly and shake them — put them down.

Relax your legs.

THE COMPLETE BREATH.

1. Sit in the cross-legged position or on a chair.
2. Draw your tummy in and exhale through your nose.
3. Let your tummy go out relaxed while inhaling through your nose, expand your ribcage and raise your chest.
4. Draw your tummy in while exhaling, your ribs move together, your chest does down.

5 X

Lie down and r e l a x.

THE LEG RAISING.

1. Lie completely relaxed, arms alongside your body.
2. Raise your right leg slowly while inhaling, *Gently stretch your heel.*
3. Lower your right leg slowly while exhaling, keep your heel stretched going down.
4. Raise your left leg while inhaling, *gently stretch your heel.*
5. Lower your left leg while exhaling, keep your heel stretched going down.

2 X

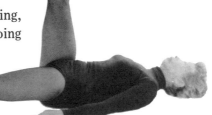

1. Put your hands under your buttocks, palms down.
2. Raise both legs slowly while inhaling, *gently stretch your heels.*
3. Lower both legs slowly while exhaling, keep your heels stretched going down.

Not for pregnant women.

2 X

The stretching of your heels also helps to stretch the hamstring muscles in back of your legs. It also is a way to get your legs gently straighter. If I should say, "try to stretch your legs," you would point your toes and get a cramp easily. Stretching the heels avoids any cramp and also gets your legs straighter. But if you feel too much stretch in back of your legs, then do not work too hard on it. It will need more time. Men especially have very tight hamstring muscles, so take it easy.

4TH WEEK.

KNEE AND HEAD RAISING.

1. Raise your arms over your head while inhaling — s t r e t c h.
2. Bring your right knee up to your chest, put your hands *and your head* to your knee — exhale.
3. Put your head down, stretch your leg down, your arms up — inhale — s t r e t c h.
4. Bring your left knee up to your chest, put your hand *and your head* to your knee — exhale.
5. Put your head down, stretch your leg down, your arms up — inhale.
6. Bring both knees up to your chest, your hands to your knees, press them down — exhale. *Don't raise your head when both knees are up.*
7. Hold the position relaxed, relieve the pressure on your knees, but keep your hands around them. Relax your back, relax your shoulders, relax your arms.
8. Put your feet down first, than stretch your legs down, your arms up — inhale — s t r e t c h.
9. Bring your arms down — exhale and r e l a x.

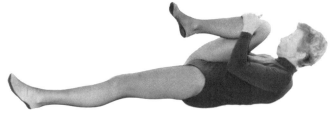

Now that your upper legs are already stretched, you can bring your knee closer to your chest, and we can put the knee and the head raising together to one movement. The important thing is just to raise your head, not

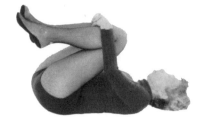

your upper body in order to get to your knee. Don't try too hard to touch your knee with your head. Just do it the easiest way. You should not feel any strain in your neck.

4TH WEEK.

KNEES OVER.

This exercise gives your back muscles and your neck muscles a gentle twist and prepares your body for the Spinal Twist. Do it gently, close your eyes and watch your body inside.

1. Lie on your back. Stretch your arms out to the sides.
2. Bend your knees, bring them close to your chest.
3. Slowly bring your knees over to your right side, turn your head s l o w l y to your left side.
4. Slowly bring your knees over to your left side, turn your head s l o w l y to your right side.

2 X

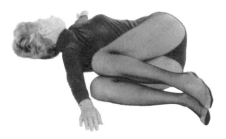

Then bring your knees up to the middle, put your feet down and relax with your knees bent, feet on the mat.

When you do this exercise, you don't have to bring your knees all the way down on your side, just go as far as you can do it relaxed. The more relaxed and stretched your back muscles get, the farther down you will be able to bring your knees, but don't force it.

NECK RELAXING MOVEMENTS.

1. Sit in cross-legged position or in chair.
2. Slowly bring your head down, chin to chest.
3. Slowly raise your head up and bring it back.

5 X

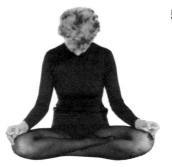
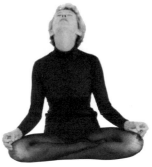

1. Slowly turn your head to your right side.
2. Slowly turn your head to your left side.

5 X

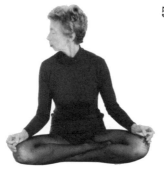
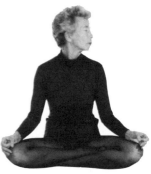

1. Slowly tilt your head toward your right shoulder.
2. Raise it up and tilt it slowly toward your left shoulder.

5 X

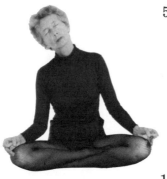
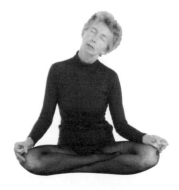

ROCK AND ROLL

1. Sit up, bend your knees, feet on mat.
2. Clasp your hands gently together under your knees.
3. Put your chin to your chest.
4. Swing your legs up gently and roll back to your shoulderblades.
5. Swing your legs down and roll up to your feet.

10 X

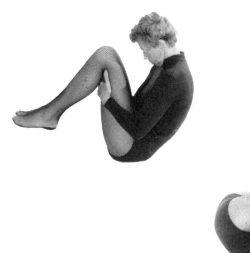
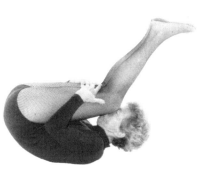

4TH WEEK.

CROSS-LEGGED ROCK AND ROLL.

Since you are now doing the first version of the Rock and Roll so well, let's go on to the next version, the Cross-legged Rock and Roll. The difference is that we roll farther back now so that your head touches the mat. But it has to be done slowly, so please follow the instructions. Caution: You have to have a good padding on the floor.

1. In the sitting position, cross your legs, hold on to your feet from the outside.
2. Lean back slightly, raise your feet about 10 inches off the mat.
3. Stretch your arms, so your feet come away from your body.
4. Slowly let yourself roll back, keep your knees bent.
5. Bring your feet fairly fast toward the crotch.
6. Let yourself roll up again.

5 X

Lie down and relax.

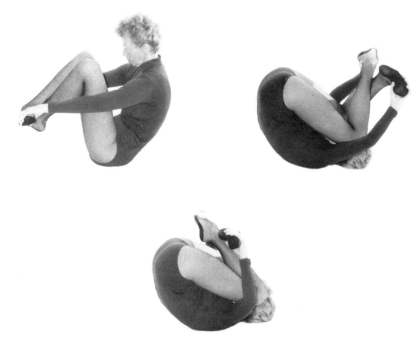

If it does not work the first time, try it again after reading the instructions carefully. The purpose is: to let yourself roll back, not to swing your legs back. You should use your body mechanics: the roundness of your back and the weight of your feet to roll back, the weight of your knees to roll up again.

Get into the starting position, and when you start rolling back don't move your muscles. They should be completely relaxed for the gentle massage they get through the rolling. When you are, for a moment, in a static stage in back, you bring your feet toward the crotch and again without moving the muscles, let yourself roll up.

How you perform this exercise depends very much on your body build. Every person is built differently, so you have to adjust the movements to your body. After a few tryouts you will find the easiest way and the most relaxed way. If you roll over too fast, do not raise your feet as high as before. If you have trouble coming up again, bring your feet faster toward the crotch. The important thing is, the rolling should be done very slowly. After a few weeks of practice you should be able to count your vertebrae when they roll up or down one by one.

4TH WEEK.

THE HALF SHOULDERSTAND.

1. Lie on your back, put your hands under your buttocks, starting with palms down.
2. Slowly raise your legs and your hips, carrying the weight of your hips on your hands.
3. Hold this position for 20 seconds. Do a gentle abdominal breathing. Keep your feet relaxed, keep your legs relaxed. Direct your consciousness to your head.
4. To come down: Lower your legs slightly farther over your head.
5. Put your hands on the mat close together.
6. Bend your knees and slowly roll your back down, bring your hips down, (they should come automatically on your hands) and stretch your legs down. R e l a x .

It is possible that you feel a slight strain in your back, not during holding the position; but the moment you lie down you feel a slight twinge in your back. If you have this feeling, then do not hold the position so long. Your back muscles need some more time to get stronger before holding the position longer. Especially practice regularly all the exercises before we get to the half shoulderstand. Never skip any of the exercises. The repetitions are the important factor in this system which strengthens your muscles. Then you can do the new exercises and the new changes easily and comfortably.

BACK-RELAXING EXERCISE.

When we follow the Half Shoulderstand with a similar backbending exercise, we first relax all the muscles in the back with the following movement.

1. Lie on your back, bring your knees high up to your chest.
2. Put your hands on your knees, fingertips pointing toward your feet.
3. Slowly bring your knees closely to your chest.
4. Then slightly to your right side.
5. As far away from your chest as your arms can reach.
6. Slightly to your left side.
7. And to your chest again.

You are making gentle circles with your knees, your hips should not roll from side to side. Close your eyes and feel how beautiful your back muscles are relaxing during this movement. *Good padding underneath.*

Repeat in the opposite direction about 5 X.

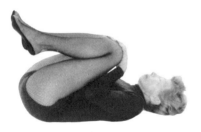

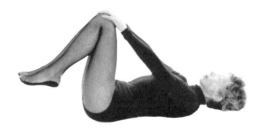

KNEE TO FOREHEAD POSE. (Preparation for Plow Posture.)

After three weeks of practice your back will be more flexible, so we are going on to the next back bending exercise, which again prepares your body for another more advanced posture.

We first go slowly into the half shoulderstand.

1. Lie on your back, put your hands under your buttocks, starting with palms down.
2. Slowly raise your legs and your hips, support them with your hands.
3. Now bring your legs slowly farther over your head, just as far as you can without feeling any strain in your neck or back.
4. Then bend your knees and put them on your forehead.
5. Hold this position for a few seconds.
6. Put your hands on the mat, keep your knees bent and slowly roll your back down, bring your hips down and stretch your legs down.

Relax.

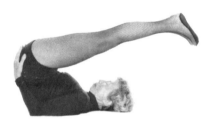 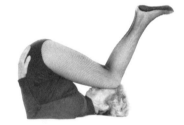

Repeat once more.

The benefits of this posture are also stretching the muscles in your back and neck, and through bringing the legs farther over, it works on increasing the blood circulation in the abdominal organs. When you put the knees on the forehead it gives a massage to the intestines and increases the peristaltic movement. It is good for constipation.

BRIDGE POSTURE.

1. Lie on your back, arms relaxed alongside your body.
2. Bend your knees, put your feet on the mat slightly apart.
3. Slowly raise your hips while inhaling. Direct your consciousness to your spine.
4. Lower your hips while exhaling, press your back down, draw your tummy in.

3 X

Relax.

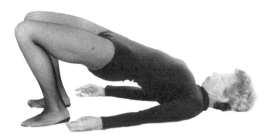

Every time you practice the bridge posture, try to raise your hips a little bit higher. Your back is getting more flexible also in this direction and again the repetition of this exercise is important to work on your muscles and to relax them, and to prepare your body for another more advanced exercise.

FORWARD BEND.

1. Sit up and spread your legs apart.
2. Slowly raise your arms at your sides over your head while inhaling.
3. Put your hands on your right knee or leg, bend down while exhaling.
4. Slide your hands up your leg, raise your arms at your sides over your head while inhaling.
5. Bend down over your left leg while exhaling.

2 X

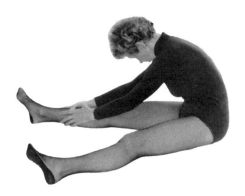

1. Put your legs together, raise your arms while inhaling.
2. Bend down over both legs while exhaling.
3. Slowly raise your body up.

2 X

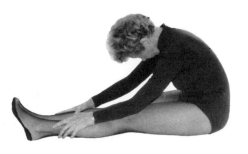

Relax your legs by shaking them gently.

SPINAL TWIST. (SECOND VERSION.)

After practicing the first version of the Spinal Twist for one week your back muscles are now stretched and more flexible. We now add another movement to the exercise by bending the stretched arm and putting it around the back. This gives a little additional twist.

1. Sit up straight, keep your right leg stretched.
2. Put your left foot over your right knee, parallel to your leg.
3. Put your right hand on your left foot.
4. Stretch your left arm forward, keep looking at your hand and slowly bring your left arm back, *then bend this arm and put it around your back.* Keep looking over your left shoulder.
5. Stretch your arm and bring it slowly forward looking at your hand. You have to unwind very slowly.
6. Put your arm down, stretch your leg, relax your legs.

Now the other side.

1. Sit up straight, keep your left leg stretched.
2. Put your right foot over your left knee, parallel to your leg.
3. Put your left hand on your right foot.
4. Stretch your right arm forward, keep looking at your hand and slowly bring your right arm back, *then bend this arm and put it around your back.* Keep looking over your right shoulder.
5. Stretch your arm and bring it slowly forward looking at your hand.
6. Put your arm down, stretch your leg, relax your legs.

Lie down and r e l a x.

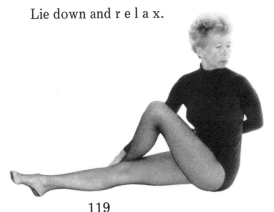

119

BACK EXERCISE. NO. 1

Even after practicing the back exercises for one whole week continue to do it very carefully and gently. The back muscles are the stiffest muscles in your body and we have to stretch them gently. *Do not do it if pregnant.*

1. Lie on your stomach, stretch your arms forward.
2. Keep stretching forward, raise your right arm, your left leg and your head while inhaling.
3. Lower arm, leg and head while exhaling.
4. Raise your left arm, your right leg and your head while inhaling.
5. Lower your arm, leg and head while exhaling.

Close your eyes during the exercise and do it very slowly watching the muscles in your back.

2 X

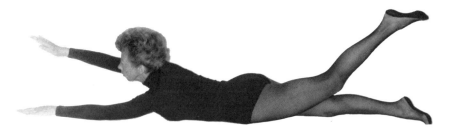

Put your hands under your chin and
r e l a x.

BACK EXERCISE NO. 2.

Strengthens the muscles in upper back and chest, firms up and slims down hips and buttocks. Gives a good posture.

1. Lie on your stomach your arms alongside your body.
2. Slowly raise your upper body, your legs and your arms while inhaling.
3. Slowly lower them while exhaling.

3 X

Only go as far as you can without feeling any strain. Always close your eyes and watch your body inside. *Do not do this exercise when pregnant.*

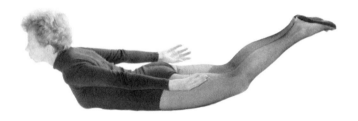

Put your hands under your chin and
r e l a x.

4TH WEEK.

LIMBERING UP KNEES AND FEET. (Preparation for Bow Posture.)

Our knee joints are built to be bent. Through sitting on chairs and sofas too much they tend to stiffen up. So any movement with them should be done carefully and relaxed and if possible without any weight pressing on them.

1. Lie on your stomach, hands under your chin.
2. Bend your knees and completely relaxed, swing your lower legs up and down, one at a time. Concentrate on relaxing your feet.

About 10 X.

If you do not feel any pain or strain, swing them a bit faster and try to touch your buttocks.

About 10 X.

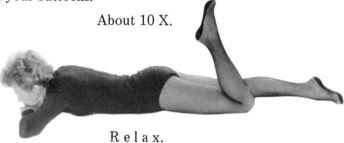

R e l a x.

THE PUSH-UPS.

1. Lie on your stomach, put your hands under your shoulders.
2. Bend your knees or keep your knees on the floor, legs stretched.
3. Push your upper body up during inhalation — slowly.
4. Lower your body during exhalation — slowly.

5 X

Relax.

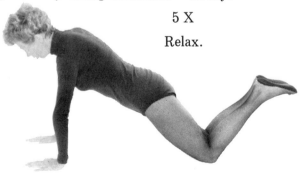

122

4TH WEEK.

YOGA MUDRA.

1. Sit back on your heels.
2. Raise your arms sideways over your head slowly while inhaling.
3. Bend forward slowly while exhaling, keep sitting on your heels, put your hands behind your back, reach for your right wrist.

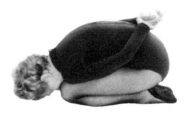

4. Put your head in the most comfortable position in front on the mat.
5. Hold the position and do a gentle abdominal breathing.
   Hold for about 10 seconds.
6. Slowly raise your body up. Go on your hands and knees. Put your feet over to one side, your hand down on the other side, sit down beside your hand, stretch your legs, relax your legs, lie down and

   r e l a x.

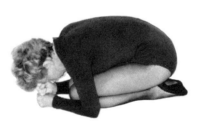

Lying down this way protects your knee cartilage from getting strained. If you just slide over from the position sitting on your heels you could easily strain the knee cartilage.

Do not do Yoga Mudra after 3rd month of pregnancy.

123

THE RELAXING POSTURE.

Close your eyes and lie in the most comfortable position. Slide your arms a few inches away from your body and turn your hands so the palms are up. When you do that the first time it does not feel as relaxed as it should, but after a few times it will relax your shoulder and upper back muscles better and you will feel very comfortable in this position.

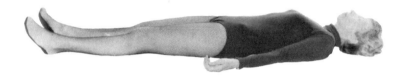

Relax your legs,
Relax your feet,
Relax your toes,
Relax your calves,
Relax your thighs,
Relax your stomach,
Relax your chest,
Relax your shoulders,
Relax your arms,
Relax your hands,
Relax your fingers,
Relax your neck,
Relax your head,
Relax your face,
Relax your mouth,
Relax your teeth,
Relax every muscle in your back.
Relax your whole body.
Relax completely;

Relax for about 10 minutes, then raise your arms over your head and s t r e t c h, roll on your left side and s t r e t c h, roll on your right side and s t r e t c h, sit up over your right side.

4TH WEEK.

SUMMARY

FOURTH WEEK'S EXERCISES.

WARM-UPS.

1.	Arm Swinging.	10 X
2.	Knee Raising.	10 X
3.	Side Bend.	3 X each side.
4.	Arm Circles.	10 X
5.	Shoulders Rolling.	5 X
6.	Squatting Down.	4 X
7.	Stretching Up.	2 X

YOGA EXERCISES.

1. Second Balancing Exercise. Hold to count of 10 each foot.
2. Wide Knee Bend and Shift. 10 X
3. Triangle Posture. Hold 5 seconds.
4. Hiprolls. 10 X each direction.
5. *Upper Leg Stretch.* 1 X each leg.
6. *Hamstring Stretch.* 2 X. Relax.
7. The Three Parts of Breathing. 5 X each.
8. Foot Exercises. 5 X each.
9. Complete Breath. 5 X
10. Leg Raising. With Stretched Heels. 2 X each.
11. Knee and Head Raising. 1 X each.
12. *Knees Over.* 2 X each side.
13. Neck Relaxing Movement. 5 X each.
14. Rock and Roll. 10 X
15. *Cross-legged Rock and Roll.* 5 X. Relax.
16. The Half Shoulderstand. Hold 20 seconds.
17. *Back Relaxing Exercise.* 5 X each direction.
18. *Knee to Forehead Pose.* (Prep. for Plow.)
19. Bridge Posture. 3 X. Relax.
20. Forward Bend. 2 X each.

4TH WEEK.

21. *Spinal Twist. (second version.)* 1 X each side. Relax.
22. *Back Exercise. No. 1 & No. 2* 2 X. Relax.
23. *Limbering Up Knees and Feet.* 10 X each.
24. The Push-Ups. 5 X. Relax.
25. Yoga Mudra. 10 seconds.
26. The Relaxing Posture. 10 minutes.

FIFTH WEEK'S EXERCISES.

Lie down and relax for a few minutes. Then sit up over your right side; stand up slowly and let's start with the Warm-Up exercises.

WARM-UPS.

1.	Arm Swinging.	10 X
2.	Knee Raising.	10 X
3.	Side Bend.	3 X
4.	Arm Circles.	10 X
5.	Shoulders Rolling.	5 X
6.	Squatting Down.	4 X
7.	Stretching Up.	2 X

FIFTH WEEK'S YOGA EXERCISES.

BALANCING EXERCISE. NO. 3.
Heel to buttock.

1. Stand on your right foot.
2. Lift your left foot up slowly.
3. Reach for your toes with your left hand.
4. Stretch your right arm up. Gently bring your heel to your buttock.
5. Hold to the count of 5.
6. Bring arm and foot down slowly.

Relax your legs, relax your shoulders.

Repeat on your left foot.

The muscles in your upper leg get stretched and your knee joints get more flexible.

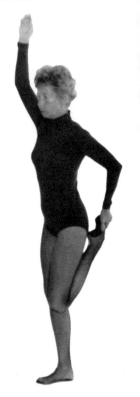

WIDE KNEE BEND AND SHIFT.

1. Put your feet wider apart than comfortable.
2. Keep your feet parallel, toes pointing straight ahead.
3. Bend your right knee, keep left leg stretched.
4. Come up, shift over and bend left knee.

10 X, count right knee.

1. Stay down and shift from side to side.

10 X, count right knee.

128

TRIANGLE POSTURE.

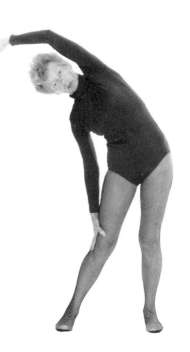

1. Put your feet comfortably apart.
2. Raise your arms, palms up, to shoulder height, while inhaling.
3. Turn your right hand around, bend down to your right side — exhale. Hold the position about 5 seconds, do a gentle abdominal breathing.
4. Slowly raise your body up, turn your hands around — inhale.
5. Bend down to your left side — exhale. Hold the position about 5 seconds, do a gentle abdominal breathing.
6. Slowly raise your body up.

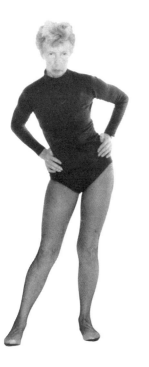

HIPROLLS.

1. Put your feet comfortably apart.
2. Put your hands on your hips.
3. Roll your hips around gently.

    10 X in each direction.

5TH WEEK.

ARMSTRETCH.

To slim down and firm up the upper arms, to stretch the shoulder and upper back muscles, to expand the chest and to give a good posture. Makes shoulder joints more flexible.

1. Put your feet slightly apart.
2. Fold your hands behind your back, *just the fingertips crossing.*
3. Raise your arms behind your back as high as you can without feeling any strain, keep your body straight.
4. Bend forward completely relaxed, keep raising your arms gently.
5. Slowly raise your body up, your arms are coming down.

Relax your arms, relax your shoulders.

2 X

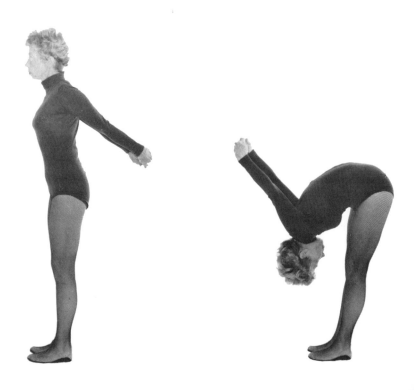

5TH WEEK.

PREPARATION FOR THE SUN EXERCISE.

UPPER LEG STRETCH.

1. Kneel down, put your hands in front of you.
2. Put your right foot forward between your hands.
3. Put your whole weight on your right foot, bring your knee forward.
4. Stretch your left leg back, resting on the knee.
5. Put your fingertips down beside your foot.
6. Raise your head gently — inhale.
7. Put your head down — exhale.
8. Bring your right knee back to your left knee, relax your legs.

   Repeat with your left leg.

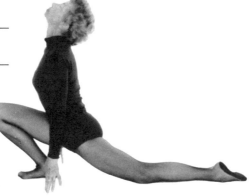

PREPARATION FOR THE SUN EXERCISE.

HAMSTRING STRETCH.

1. Kneel down, put your hands in front of you.
2. Curl in your toes and stretch your legs.
3. Keep feet and hands where they are.
4. Gently and carefully bring your heels down a little bit.
5. Kneel down and relax your legs.

2 X

Put your feet over to one side, sit down on the other side. Stretch your legs, relax your legs, lie down and
r e l a x.

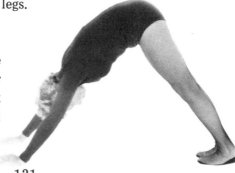

5TH WEEK.

THE BREATHING EXERCISES.

THE ABDOMINAL BREATHING.

1. Sit cross-legged or on a chair, put your hands on your tummy.
2. Draw your tummy in — exhale.
3. Let your tummy go out completely relaxed — inhale.
4. Draw your tummy in — exhale.

5 X

THE MIDDLE OR RIBCAGE BREATHING.

1. Sit cross-legged or on a chair, put your hands on your ribcage.
2. Squeeze your ribs gently together — exhale.
3. Expand your ribcage — inhale.
4. Feel your ribs moving together — exhale.

5 X

THE UPPER OR CHEST BREATHING.

1. Sit cross-legged or on a chair, put your fingertips on your collarbones.
2. Exhale through your nose, feel your chest going down.
3. Inhale slowly by raising your chest, expanding your shoulders.
4. Exhale, feel your chest going down.

5 X

Stretch your legs, relax your legs by shaking them gently.

This time we did not relax and shake the legs after each breathing exercise, because your legs slowly are getting used to being in the cross-legged position a bit longer without any strain. But the moment you start feeling uncomfortable, just stretch your legs and relax them. Try to sit in the cross-legged position as often as possible. It strengthens the tendons and muscles in the abdominal area and is *especially beneficial during pregnancy and afterwards.*

5TH WEEK.

FOOT EXERCISES.

1. In the sitting position put your hands behind you.
2. Stretch your feet, but don't point your toes, stretch your instep.
3. Stretch your heels, feel a gentle stretch in back of your calves.

5 X

1. Spread your legs slightly apart.
2. Roll your feet around in gentle circles.
3. Roll them in the opposite directions slowly and relaxed.

5 X in each direction

1. Raise your right leg slightly and shake it — put it down.
2. Raise your left leg slightly and shake it — put it down.
3. Raise both legs slightly and shake them — put them down.

Relax your legs.

THE COMPLETE BREATH.

1. Sit in the cross-legged position or on a chair.
2. Draw your tummy in and exhale through your nose.
3. Let your tummy go out relaxed while inhaling through your nose, expand your ribcage and raise your chest, while inhaling through your nose.
4. Draw your tummy in, your ribs go together, your chest goes down while exhaling.

5 X

Lie down and r e l a x .

5TH WEEK.

THE LEG RAISING.

1. Lie completely relaxed, arms alongside your body.
2. Raise your right leg slowly while inhaling, gently stretch your heel.
3. Lower your right leg slowly while exhaling, keep your heel stretched while going down.
4. Raise your left leg while inhaling, gently stretch your heel.
5. Lower your left leg while exhaling, keep your heel stretched going down.

2 X

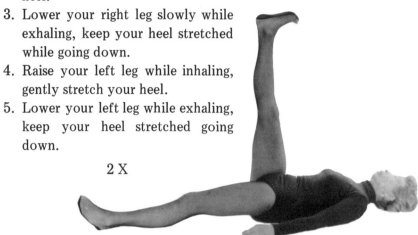

1. Put your hands under your buttocks, palms down.
2. Raise both legs slowly while inhaling, gently stretch your heels.
3. Lower both legs slowly while exhaling, keep your heels stretched going down.

   Not for pregnant women.

2 X

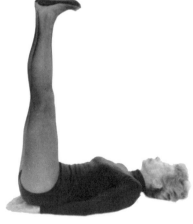

KNEE AND HEAD RAISING.

1. Raise your arms over your head while inhaling — s t r e t c h.
2. Bring your right knee up to your chest, put your hands and your head to your knee — exhale.
3. Put your head down, stretch your leg down, your arms up — inhale s t r e t c h.
4. Bring your left knee up to your chest, put your hands and your head to your knee — exhale.
5. Put your head down, stretch your leg down, your arms up — inhale.
6. Bring both knees up to your chest, your hands to your knees, press them down — exhale. Don't raise your head when both knees are up.
7. Hold the position relaxed, relieve the pressure on your knees, but keep your hands around them. Relax your back, relax your arms, relax your shoulders.
8. Put your feet down first, then stretch your legs down, your arms up inhale — s t r e t c h.
9. Bring your arms down — exhale and r e l a x.

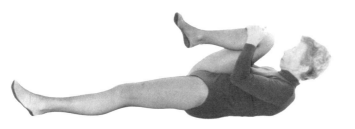

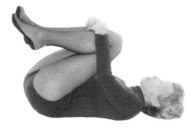

5TH WEEK.

LEG UP AND DOWN.

Your abdominal and back muscles are stronger now, so we are going to do a leg exercise which puts slightly more demand on your muscles. *Not for pregnant women.*

1. Lie on your back, put your hands under your buttocks, palms down.
2. Raise your right leg straight up.
3. Raise your left leg up and at the same time bring your right leg down. They both move at the same time.
4. Raise your right leg, bring your left leg down.
5. Raise your left leg, bring your right leg down.

10 X, count right leg.

Lie down and r e l a x .

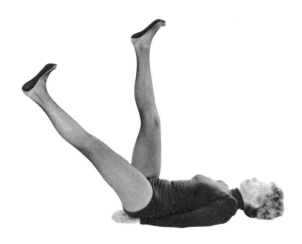

5TH WEEK.

NECK RELAXING MOVEMENTS.

1. Sit in cross-legged position or on chair.
2. Slowly bring your head down, chin toward chest.
3. Slowly raise your head up and bring it back.

5 X

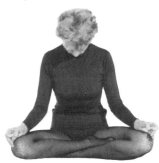
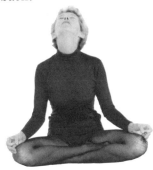

1. Slowly turn your head to your right side.
2. Slowly turn your head to your left side.

5 X

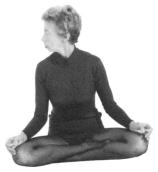
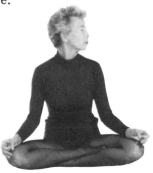

1. Slowly tilt your head toward your right shoulder.
2. Raise it up and tilt it slowly toward your left shoulder.

5 X

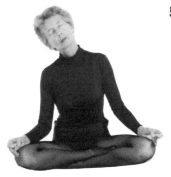
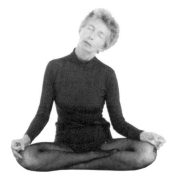

ROCK AND ROLL.

1. Sit up, bend your knees, feet on mat.
2. Clasp your hands gently together under your knees.
3. Put your chin to your chest.
4. Swing your legs up gently and roll back to your shoulderblades.
5. Swing your legs down and roll up to your feet.

10 X

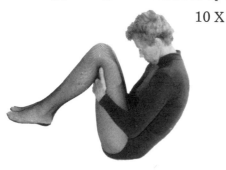
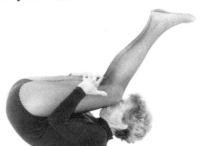

CROSS-LEGGED ROCK AND ROLL.

1. Sit up, cross your legs, hold on to your feet from the outside.
2. Lean back slightly, raise your feet about 10 inches off the mat.
3. Stretch your arms, so your feet get away from your body.
4. Slowly let yourself roll back, keep your knees bent.
5. Bring your feet fairly fast toward the crotch.
6. Let yourself roll up again.

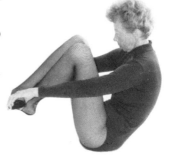

5 X

Lie down and relax.

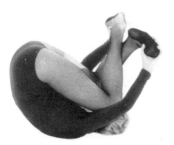
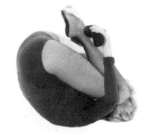

138

THE HALF SHOULDERSTAND.

1. Lie on your back, put your hands under your buttocks, starting with palms down.
2. Slowly raise your legs and your hips, carry the weight of your hips on your hands.
3. Hold this position for 25 seconds. Do a gentle abdominal breathing. Keep your feet relaxed, keep your legs relaxed.
4. To come down: Lower your feet slightly farther over your head.
5. Put your hands on the mat close together.
6. Bend your knees and slowly roll your back down, bring your hips down, (they should come automatically on your hands), and stretch your legs down.
   Lie down and r e l a x .

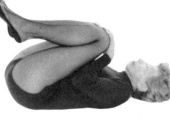

BACK RELAXING EXERCISE.

1. Lie on your back, bring your knees high up to your chest.
2. Put your hands on your knees, fingertips pointing toward your feet.
3. Slowly bring your knees closer to your chest.
4. Then slightly to your right side.
5. As far away from your chest as your arms can reach.
6. Slightly to your left side.
7. And to your chest again.

       5 X in each direction.

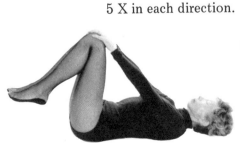

5TH WEEK.

KNEE TO FOREHEAD POSE. (Preparation for Plow Posture.)

We first go into the Half Shoulderstand.

1. Lie on your back, put your hands under your buttocks, starting with palms down.
2. Slowly raise your legs and hips, support them with your hands.
3. Now bring your legs slowly farther over your head, just as far as you can without feeling any strain in your neck or back.
4. Then bend your knees and put them on your forehead.
5. Hold this position for a few seconds.
6. Put your hands on the mat, keep your knees bent and slowly roll your back down, bring your hips down and stretch your legs down.

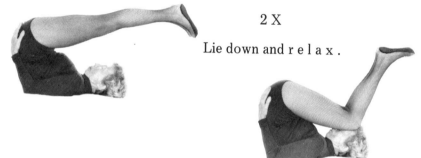

2 X

Lie down and r e l a x .

BRIDGE POSTURE.

1. Lie on your back, arms relaxed alongside your body.
2. Bend your knees, put your feet on the mat slightly apart.
3. Slowly raise your hips while inhaling.
4. Lower your hips while exhaling, press your back down, draw your tummy in.

3 X

Lie down and r e l a x .

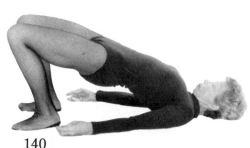

5TH WEEK.

FORWARD BEND.

1. Sit up and spread your legs apart.
2. Slowly raise your arms at your sides over your head while inhaling.
3. Put your hands on your right knee or leg, bend down while exhaling.
4. Slide your hands up your leg, raise your arms at your sides over your head while inhaling.
5. Bend down over your left leg while exhaling.

2 X

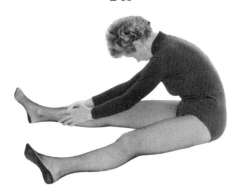

1. Put your legs together, raise your arms while inhaling.
2. Bend down over both legs while exhaling.

2 X

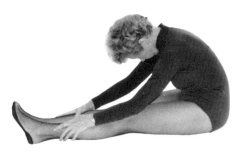

Relax your legs by shaking them gently.

5TH WEEK.

REST OF AN ANIMAL.

A very nice relaxing posture which works only on your upper leg muscles and relaxes your whole body.

1. Sit up, spread your legs apart.
2. Put the sole of your right foot against the inside of your left thigh.
3. Put your left foot behind your left thigh.
4. Raise your arms over your head while inhaling.
5. Bend down over your *right* knee while exhaling, put your head down and relax in this position, do a gentle abdominal breathing.
6. Slowly raise your head, slide your hands over the mat, raise your arms over your head while inhaling.
7. Bend down again over your right knee while exhaling. Relax.
8. Raise your head up, slide your hands over the mat. Put them behind you, lean back a little, stretch your legs, relax your legs.

Repeat on the other side.

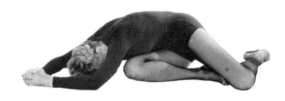

5TH WEEK.

CRAWLING. (On the carpet on all fours.)

1. Get on your hands and knees.
2. Put your right knee and your left hand forward.
3. Put your left knee and your right hand forward. Keep doing this with small steps all around the room.

Start with one round and increase the crawling time slowly over the months to 20 minutes. It can be done at any time of the day. It does not have to be connected with the Yoga session, but would be good to include it.

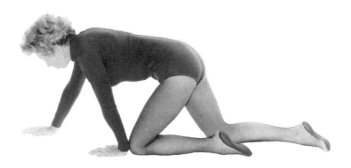

Through doing push-ups regularly your wrists, arms and shoulders are strong enough to do this delightful exercise, which will benefit every part of your body. It strengthens wrists, arms, shoulders, neck and back muscles, also leg and stomach muscles. And it helps your brain to work better.

It is an exercise which comes naturally. Every baby wants to do it in the sequence of his development to strengthen his muscles and to develop his brain. Unfortunately many mothers don't know how important this crawling period in the life of their baby is. They deprive their children of this crawling period fearing that they could get dirty. They put them in walkers or jumpers, which force the children to activities too advanced for their muscle strength. The development of the muscles has to go slowly in the way nature designed it. If we fool with mother nature we have to pay for it. Research showed that children who have reading problems in school are the ones who were deprived of their crawling period during babyhood.

We have tried to remedy this by crawling with children of all ages, even to college age. It has shown that their brain can still benefit from this. Their comprehension gets better, the ability to think and the memory improve. And especially so does the strength of their back muscles, which are also very weak in children who did not crawl as babies.

In one of my Yoga Teachers' Courses we heard one mother telling us about her son who is a gifted child. To bring all his potentials out, their doctor recommended crawling twice a day for 20 minutes. Now the whole family is crawling.

Now you start crawling too. It will not be easy in the beginning, so start with one round in your living room; stay on the carpet. If it feels uncomfortable on your knees, get some knee pads (at garden supply stores).

The benefits lie in the gentle moving of the whole body — stretching and relaxing the spine. It is especially good for your back. If you can do it for 10-20 minutes it also works on your cardio-vascular system.

I read somewhere that one of those big business tycoons is crawling around every morning before he starts working and he claims that it keeps his body and mind young.

After crawling lie down and relax. Take a few complete breaths. Concentrate on the exhalation and feel how every part of your body relaxes.

THE RELAXING POSTURE.

Close your eyes and lie in the most comfortable position.

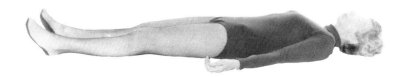

Relax your legs.
Relax your feet.
Relax your toes.
Relax your calves.
Relax your thighs.
Relax your stomach.
Relax your chest.
Relax your shoulders.
Relax your arms.
Relax your hands.
Relax your fingers.
Relax your neck.
Relax your head.
Relax your face.
Relax your mouth.
Relax your teeth.
Relax every muscle in your back.
Relax your whole body.
Relax completely.

Relax for about 10 minutes. Then raise your arms over your head and stretch, roll on your left side and stretch, roll on your right side and stretch, sit up over your right side.

Thank you, see you tomorrow.

SUMMARY

FIFTH WEEK'S EXERCISES.

WARM-UPS.

1.	Arm Swinging.	10 X
2.	Knee Raising.	10 X
3.	Side Bend.	3 X each side.
4.	Arm Circles.	10 X
5.	Shoulders Rolling.	5 X
6.	Squatting Down.	4 X
7.	Stretching Up.	2 X

YOGA EXERCISES.

1. Balancing Exercise No. 3. Hold to count of 5 on each foot.
2. Wide Knee Bend and Shift. 10 X
3. Triangle Posture. Hold 5 seconds.
4. Hiprolls. 10 X each direction.
5. *Armstretch.* 2 X
6. Upper Leg Stretch. 1 X each leg.
7. Hamstring Stretch. 2 X
8. The Three Parts of Breathing. 5 X each.
9. Foot Exercises. 5 X each.
10. The Complete Breath. 5 X
11. The Leg Raising. 2 X each.
12. Knee and Head Raising. 1 X each. Relax.
13. *Leg Up and Down.* 10 X each leg. Relax.
14. Neck Relaxing Movement. 5 X each.
15. Rock and Roll. 10 X
16. Cross-legged Rock and Roll. 5 X. Relax.
17. The Half Shoulderstand. Hold 25 seconds.
18. Back Relaxing Exercise. 5 X each direction.
19. Knee to Forehead Pose. 2 X. Relax.
20. Bridge Posture. 3 X. Relax.

21. Forward Bend. 2 X each.
22. *Rest of an Animal.* 1 X each side.
23. *Crawling.*
24. The Relaxing Posture. 10 minutes.

SIXTH WEEK'S EXERCISES.

Lie down and relax for a few minutes. Then sit up over your right side; stand up slowly and let's start with the Warm-Up exercises.

WARM-UPS.

1.	Arm Swinging.	10 X
2.	Knee Raising.	10 X
3.	Side Bend.	3 X
4.	Arm Circles.	10 X
5.	Shoulders Rolling.	5 X
6.	Squatting Down.	4 X
7.	Stretching Up.	2 X

6TH WEEK.

SIXTH WEEK'S YOGA EXERCISES.

BALANCING EXERCISE NO. 4. Scale.

1. Stand on your right foot.
2. Stretch your arms out to the sides.
3. Lean forward slightly.
4. Raise your left leg in back.
5. Concentrate on a spot about 3 feet in front of you.
6. Hold for 10 seconds.

Repeat standing on left foot.

Relax your legs by shaking them.

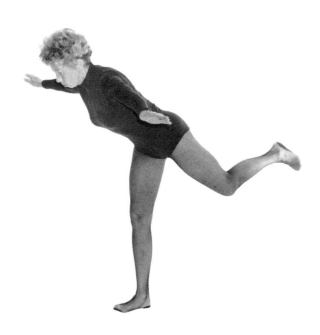

6TH WEEK.

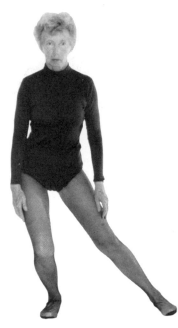

WIDE KNEE BEND AND SHIFT.

1. Put your feet wider apart than is comfortable.
2. Keep your feet parallel, toes pointing straight ahead.
3. Bend your right knee, keep left leg stretched.
4. Come up, shift over and bend left knee.

   10 X count right knee.

1. Stay down and shift from side to side.

   10 X count right knee.

TRIANGLE POSTURE.

1. Put your feet comfortably apart.
2. Raise your arms, palms up, to shoulder height, while inhaling.
3. Turn your right hand around, bend down to your right side — exhale. Hold the position about 5 seconds, do a gentle abdominal breathing.
4. Slowly raise your body up, turn your hands around — inhale.
5. Bend down to your left side — exhale.
   Hold the position about 5 seconds, do a gentle abdominal breathing.
6. Slowly raise your body up.

   Relax your legs.

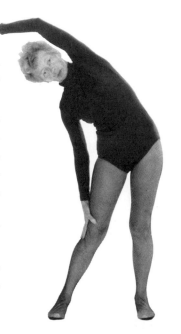

150

6TH WEEK.

HIPROLLS.

1. Put your feet comfortably apart.
2. Put your hands on your hips.
3. Roll your hips around gently.

        10 X in each direction.

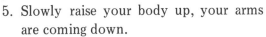

ARMSTRETCH.

1. Put your feet comfortably apart.
2. Fold your hands behind your back, just fingertips crossing.
3. Raise your arms behind your back as high as you can without feeling any strain, keep your body straight.

    4. Bend forward completely relaxed, keep raising your arms.

      5. Slowly raise your body up, your arms are coming down.

      Relax your arms, relax your shoulders.

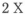

2 X

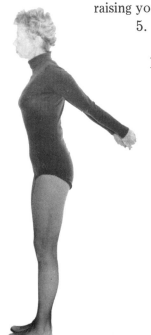

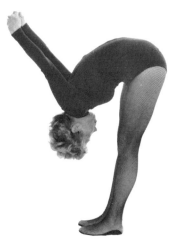

6TH WEEK.

PREPARATIONS FOR THE SUN EXERCISE.

UPPER LEG STRETCH.

1. Kneel down, put your hands in front of you.
2. Put your right foot forward between your hands.
3. Put your whole weight on your right foot, bring your knee forward.
4. Stretch your left leg back, resting on the knee.
5. Put your fingertips down beside your foot.
6. Raise your head gently — inhale.
7. Put your head down — exhale.
8. Bring your right knee back to your left knee, relax your legs.

Repeat with your left leg.

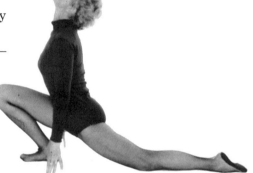

HAMSTRING STRETCH.

1. Kneel down, put your hands in front of you.
2. Curl in your toes and stretch your legs.
3. Keep feet and hands where they are.
4. Gently and carefully bring your heels down a little bit.
5. Kneel down and relax your legs.

2 X

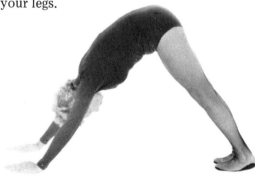

PREPARATION FOR THE SUN EXERCISE.

THE STEP FORWARD.

1. Kneel down, put your hands in front of you.
2. Curl in your toes and stretch your legs.
3. Bring your right foot forward between your hands.
4. Stretch your right knee forward, your left leg back resting on knee.
5. Bring your right knee back to your left knee, relax your legs.

Repeat with left foot forward.

It is not an easy exercise for a lot of people, so keep practicing. It will help, if you concentrate on keeping your hips high up until you put your foot down in front.

It is part of a sequence of exercises, we are going to learn next week.

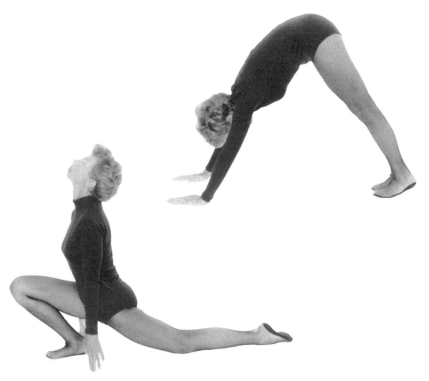

6TH WEEK.

THE BREATHING EXERCISES (Pranayama called in sanskrit).

THE ABDOMINAL BREATHING.

1. Sit in cross-legged position or on a chair, put your hands on your tummy.
2. Draw your tummy in — exhale.
3. Let your tummy go out relaxed — inhale.
4. Draw your tummy in — exhale.

5 X

THE MIDDLE OR RIBCAGE BREATHING.

1. Sit cross-legged or on a chair, put your hands on your ribcage.
2. Squeeze your ribs gently together — exhale.
3. Expand your ribcage — inhale.
4. Feel your ribs moving together — exhale.

5 X

THE UPPER OR CHEST BREATHING.

1. Sit cross-legged or on a chair, put your fingertips on your collarbones.
2. Exhale, feel your chest going down.
3. Inhale slowly, feel your chest raising, your shoulders expanding.
4. Exhale, feel your chest going down.

5 X

Relax your legs.

6TH WEEK.

FOOT EXERCISES.

1. In the sitting position put your hands behind you.
2. Stretch your feet, but don't point your toes, stretch your instep.
3. Stretch your heels, feel a gentle stretch in back of your calves.

5 X

1. Spread your legs slightly apart.
2. Roll your feet around in gentle circles.
3. Roll them in the opposite directions slowly and relaxed.

5 X

1. Raise your right leg slightly and shake it — put it down.
2. Raise your left leg slightly and shake it — put it down.
3. Raise both legs slightly and shake them — put them down.

Relax your legs.

6TH WEEK.

THE COMPLETE BREATH.

After practicing The Complete Breath for several weeks, we will do it now with counting.

1. Draw your tummy in — exhale.
2. Let your tummy go out, expand your ribcage and raise your chest while inhaling to the count of 8.
3. Draw your tummy in, your ribs go together, your chest goes down while exhaling to the count of 8.
4. There are 3 counts of rest, then inhale again.

5 X

There are 3 counts of rest, because when you take a deep breath like that, you don't have to inhale right away again.

The rhythm of your counting depends on your life rhythm. The Yogis in India take their pulse beat and use this for their counting rhythm, and you can do that too.

Turn your right hand around, palm up, put the fingertips of your left hand above your right wrist on the side where the thumb is and feel your pulse beat. Listen to it, count with it and get your own personal rhythm for your breathing exercises. Everything in your body works rhythmically, so also your breathing.

If the count of 8 should feel too long, change it to 6. When your lung capacity grows you will be able to do it with the count of 8.

Important is: Never hold your breath. You should feel comfortable while doing the breathing exercises. Don't work hard on it.

6TH WEEK.

THE LEG RAISING.

1. Lie completely relaxed, arms alongside your body.
2. Raise your right leg slowly while inhaling, gently stretch your heel.
3. Lower your right leg slowly while exhaling, keep your heel stretched going down.
4. Raise your left leg while inhaling, gently stretch your heel.
5. Lower your left leg while exhaling, keep your heel stretched going down.

2 X

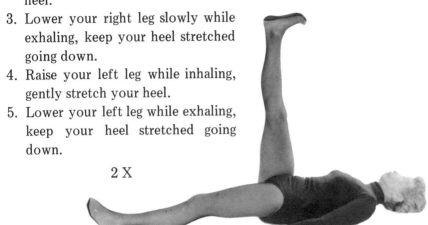

1. Put your hands under your buttocks, palms down.
2. Raise both legs slowly while inhaling, gently stretch your heels.
3. Lower both legs down while exhaling, keep heels stretched going down. *Not for pregnant women.*

2 X

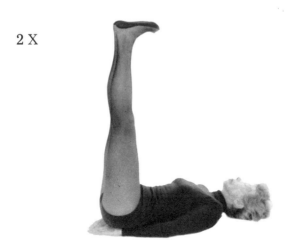

KNEE AND HEAD RAISING.

1. Raise your arms over your head while inhaling — stretch.
2. Bring your right knee up to your chest, put your hands and your head to your knee — exhale.
3. Put your head down, stretch your leg down, your arms up — inhale — stretch.
4. Bring your left knee up to your chest, put your hands and your head to your knee — exhale.
5. Put your head down, stretch your leg down, your arms up — inhale.
6. Bring both knees up to your chest, your hands to your knees, press them down — exhale.
7. Hold the position relaxed, relieve the pressure on your knees, but keep your hands around them. Relax your back, relax your arms, relax your shoulders.
8. Put your feet down first, then stretch your legs down, your arms up — inhale — stretch.
9. Bring your arms down — exhale and relax.

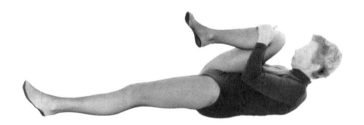

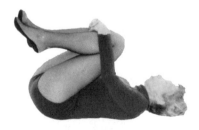

6TH WEEK.

BOTH LEGS DOWN SLOWLY.

This week we will do again an exercise which really works on your abdominal muscles. But they have to have a certain strength already. Watch it carefully. If you feel it is too much for your muscles, just stop after 2 or 3 times and relax.

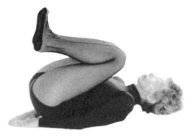

1. Put your hands under your buttocks, palms down.
2. Bring both knees high up to your chest.
3. Stretch both legs straight up and s l o w l y lower them down to about 5 inches from the mat.
4. Bend your legs, bring your knees high up to your chest and start again.

3-5 X

The beauty of this exercise is the change from working with the abdominal muscles and relaxing them. When you lower the legs slowly, your muscles are working, when you bend your knees and bring them high up to the chest, the muscles are relaxing. Close your eyes and feel this movement and this change inside.

Don't do it if pregnant.

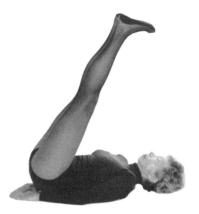

NECK RELAXING MOVEMENTS.

1. Sit in cross-legged position or on chair.
2. Slowly bring your head down, chin toward chest.
3. Slowly raise your head up and bring it back.

5 X

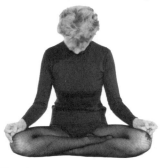 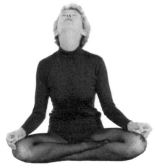

1. Slowly turn your head to your right side.
2. Slowly turn your head to your left side.

5 X

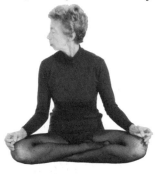 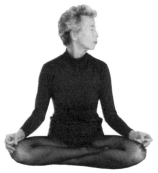

1. Slowly tilt your head toward your right shoulder.
2. Raise it up and tilt it slowly toward your left shoulder.

5 X

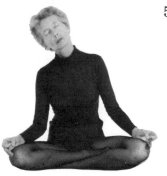 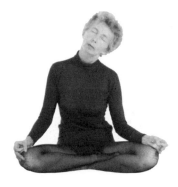

6TH WEEK.

ROCK AND ROLL.

1. Sit up, bend your knees, feet on mat.
2. Clasp your hands gently together under your knees.
3. Put your chin to your chest.
4. Swing your legs up gently and roll back to your shoulder blades.
5. Swing your legs down and roll up to your feet.

10 X

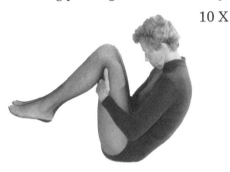 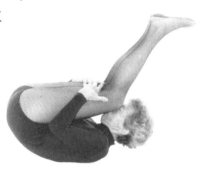

CROSS-LEGGED ROCK AND ROLL.

1. Sit up, cross your legs, hold on to your feet from the outside.
2. Lean back slightly, raise your feet about 10 inches off the mat.
3. Stretch your arms, so your feet get away from your body.
4. Slowly let yourself roll back, keep your knees bent.
5. Bring your feet fairly fast toward the crotch.
6. Let yourself roll up again.

5 X

Lie down and relax.

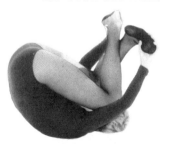 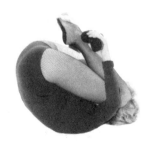

6TH WEEK.

THE HALF SHOULDERSTAND.

1. Lie on your back, put your hands under your buttocks, starting with palms down.
2. Slowly raise your legs and hips, carry the weight of your hips on your hands.
3. Hold this position as long as you can, easily and relaxed. Do a gentle abdominal breathing, direct your consciousness to your face and head. Look inside and feel the blood circulating better in the parts where your consciousness is directed. But the moment you start feeling uncomfortable stop holding the position.
4. Lower your feet slightly farther over your head.
5. Put your hands on the mat close together.
6. Bend your knees and slowly roll your back down, bring your hips down, they should come automatically on your hands, and stretch your legs down.

Lie there completely r e l a x e d.

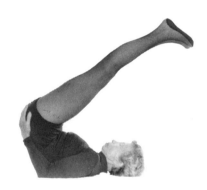

6TH WEEK.

BACK RELAXING EXERCISE.

1. Lie on your back, bring your knees high up to your chest.
2. Put your hands on your knees, fingertips pointing toward your feet.
3. Slowly bring your knees closer to your chest.
4. Then slightly to your right side.
5. As far away from your chest as your arms can reach.
6. Slightly to your left side.
7. And to your chest again. Close your eyes and direct your consciousness to the muscles in your back.

5 X in each direction.

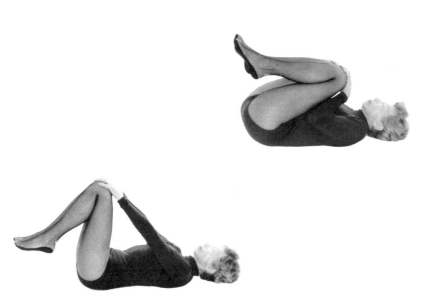

KNEE TO FOREHEAD POSE. (Preparation for Plow Posture.)

We are going first into the Half Shoulderstand.

1. Lie on your back, put your hands under your buttocks, starting with palms down.
2. Slowly raise your legs and hips, support them with your hands.
3. Now bring your legs slowly farther over your head, only as far as you can without feeling any strain in your neck or back, or pressure in your head.
4. Then bend your knees and put them on your forehead.
5. Hold this position for a few seconds.
6. Put your hands on the mat, keep your knees bent and slowly roll your back down, bring your hips down and stretch your legs down.

2 X

Lie down and r e l a x.

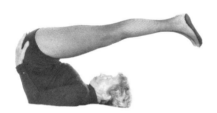 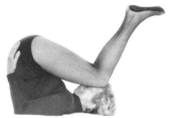

Every time you practice this position you will feel that your legs come farther down over your head because your neck and your back are getting more flexible, but do not force them down. One day when you can touch your toes to the mat easily and relaxed and can keep your legs stretched doing it, you will have accomplished the Plow Posture, a beautiful but more advanced Yoga exercise. Some people can do this exercise easily from the beginning, some can do it after weeks or years of practice, some will never be able to do it; it also depends very much on the body build. Just bringing the legs over as far as possible without any strain gives the same benefits. *The important thing is: always limber up the neck first with the Neck Movements, the Rock and Roll, the Half Shoulderstand before going into the Plow or into the Knee to Forehead Pose.*

6TH WEEK.

BRIDGE POSTURE.

1. Lie on your back, arms relaxed alongside your body.
2. Bend your knees, put your feet on the mat slightly apart.
3. Slowly raise your hips while inhaling.
4. Lower your hips while exhaling, press your back down, draw your tummy in.

3 X

R e l a x.

By now you know very well the muscles which work in your body during this exercise, so from now on try to concentrate on your spine. Close your eyes, and vertebra by vertebra, roll your spine up and also slowly roll it down again. Feel every part rolling down, press it down. This way your spine will get a beautiful massage. Feel yourself into your spine and you will enjoy this exercise more and more every time.

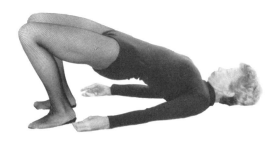

FORWARD BEND.

1. Sit up and spread your legs apart.
2. Slowly raise your arms at your sides over your head while inhaling.
3. Bend down over your right leg while exhaling.
4. Raise your arms at your sides over your head while inhaling.
5. Bend down over your left leg while exhaling.

2 X

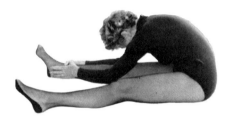

1. Put your legs together, raise your arms at your sides over your head while inhaling.
2. Bend down over both legs while exhaling.

2 X

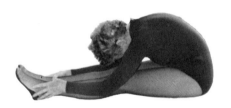

Relax your legs by shaking them gently.

Try to do this exercise more slowly each time. Close your eyes and watch your muscles inside. You will also get more flexible step by step in this movement. Even if you sometimes feel like you are not progressing, it will take time so just be patient. You get the benefits of this movement in any case.

6TH WEEK.

BACK EXERCISE NO. 1.

1. Lie on your stomach, stretch your arms forward.
2. Keep stretching forward, raise your right arm, your left leg and your head while inhaling.
3. Lower arm, leg and head while exhaling.
4. Raise your left arm, your right leg and your head while inhaling.
5. Lower your arm, leg and head while exhaling.

2 X

Put your hands under your chin and r e l a x.

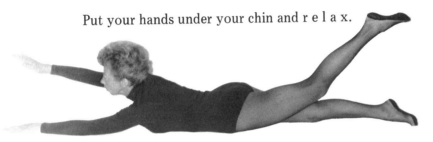

Do not do this exercise when pregnant.

BACK EXERCISE NO. 2.

Strengthens the muscles in the upper back and chest, firms up and slims down hips and buttocks. Gives a good posture.

1. Lie on your stomach, arms alongside your body.
2. Slowly raise your upper body, your legs and your arms while inhaling.
3. Slowly lower them while exhaling.

3 X

Only go as far as you can without feeling any strain. Always close your eyes and watch your body inside. *Do not do this exercise when pregnant.*

6TH WEEK.

PREPARATION FOR COBRA POSTURE.

This movement is especially to let you feel which muscles to watch when we start doing the Cobra Posture.

1. Lie on your stomach, put your hands under your shoulders, fingertips pointing forward.
2. Put your forehead on the mat.
3. Very slowly raise your head while inhaling (just your head).
4. Slowly lower your head while exhaling.

2 X

You will feel the muscles in the middle of your back. It should be a gentle stretch not a strain. Just by bringing your head up and back, these muscles are working, and these are the muscles which you should watch during the Cobra Posture. If you did not feel these muscles in your back, then your neck muscles are not yet flexible enough to bring the back muscles into action. Practicing the neck movements every day 4-5 X will help to relieve the tension in the neck and will make it more flexible.

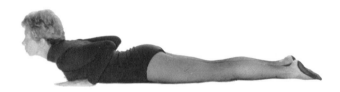

6TH WEEK.

THE COBRA.

Stretches the muscles in chest, abdominal area, strengthens back muscles. Slims down and firms up tummy, buttocks and upper legs. Stretches neck and chin area. Increases blood circulation in liver, spleen, kidneys.

1. Lie on your stomach, put your hands under your shoulders, fingertips pointing forward.
2. Put your forehead on the mat, spread your feet slightly apart.
3. During inhalation slowly raise your head, raise your upper body without helping with your arms, just supporting.
4. During exhalation slowly lower your body, the last part to come down is your head.

2 X

The most important task in this posture is: to do it very slowly and feel your body. Slowly roll your body up; the region below the navel should stay on the mat, so your arms are always bent slightly. Also very slowly roll your body down again. One of the most beautiful movements in the Yoga exercise system. *Not for pregnant women.*

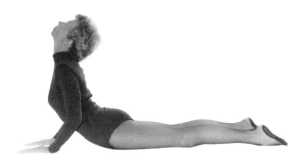

6TH WEEK.

YOGA MUDRA.

The Yoga Mudra position feels especially good after doing the Cobra. It relaxes and stretches all the muscles in the back we just worked with. If you feel even the slightest strain in your back, then do a gentle abdominal breathing during the Yoga Mudra posture and watch your back breathe. During exhalation these back muscles relax beautifully.

1. Sit back on your heels.
2. Raise your arms sideways over your head slowly while inhaling.
3. Slowly bend forward while exhaling, keep sitting on your heels, put your hands behind your back, reach for your right wrist.
4. Put your head in the most comfortable position in front on the mat.
5. Hold the position and do a gentle abdominal breathing, feel your back muscles relax. Hold as long as you feel comfortable.
6. Slowly raise your body up. Get on your hands and knees. Put your feet over to one side, sit down on the other side, stretch your legs, relax your legs, lie down and r e l a x.

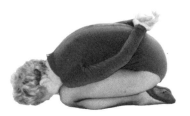

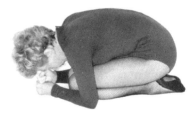

6TH WEEK.

CRAWLING. (On all fours on the carpet.)

1. Get on hands and knees.
2. Bring your right knee and your left hand forward.
3. Bring your left knee and your right hand forward.

Keep doing this twice around the room. Do it gently and relaxed. Think about all the benefits you get from these movements. Get your whole family to do it.

Lie down and relax.

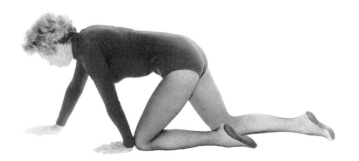

6TH WEEK.

THE RELAXING POSTURE.

Close your eyes and lie in the most comfortable position. Arms slightly away from your body. Palms turned up. Shoulders relaxed.

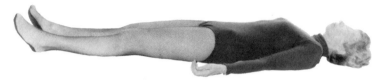

Relax your legs.
Relax your feet.
Relax your toes.
Relax your calves.
Relax your thighs.
Relax your stomach.
Relax your chest.
Relax your shoulders.
Relax your arms.
Relax your hands.
Relax your fingers.
Relax your neck.
Relax your head.
Relax your face.
Relax your mouth.
Relax your teeth.
Relax every muscle in your back.
Relax your whole body.
Relax completely.

Relax for about 10 minutes. Then raise your arms over your head and s t r e t c h, roll on your left side and s t r e t c h, roll on your right side and s t r e t c h. Sit up over your right side.

Thank you, see you tomorrow.

6TH WEEK.

SUMMARY

SIXTH WEEK'S EXERCISES.

WARM-UPS.

1.	Arm Swinging.	10 X
2.	Knee Raising.	10 X
3.	Side Bend.	3 X each side.
4.	Arm Circles.	10 X
5.	Shoulders Rolling.	5 X
6.	Squatting Down.	4 X
7.	Stretching Up.	2 X

YOGA EXERCISES.

1. *Balancing Exercise No. 4.* Scale. Hold 10 seconds. 1 X each foot.
2. Wide Knee Bend and Shift. 10 X
3. Triangle Posture. 5 seconds.
4. Hiprolls. 10 X each direction.
5. Armstretch. 2 X
6. Upper Leg Stretch. 1 X each leg.
7. Hamstring Stretch. 2 X
8. *The Step Forward.* 1 X each foot.
9. The Breathing Exercises. 5 X each.
10. The Foot Exercises. 5 X each.
11. The Complete Breath. 5 X. Relax.
12. The Leg Raising. 2 X each. Relax.
13. Knee and Head Raising. 1 X each. Relax.
14. *Both Legs Down Slowly.* 3-5 X
15. Neck Relaxing Movements. 5 X each.
16. Rock and Roll. 10 X
17. Cross-legged Rock and Roll. 5 X. Relax.
18. The Half Shoulderstand. Hold as long as comfortable.
19. Back Relaxing Exercise. 5 X each direction.
20. Knee to Forehead Pose. 2 X. Relax.

6TH WEEK.

21. Bridge Posture. 3 X. Relax.
22. Forward Bend. 2 X each. Relax.
23. Back Exercises No. 1 2 X. Relax.
24. Back Exercise No. 2 3 X. Relax.
25. *Preparation for Cobra Posture.* 2 X. Relax.
26. *The Cobra Posture.* 2 X.
27. Yoga Mudra.
28. Crawling. (2 rounds in your living room.)
29. The Relaxing Posture.

SEVENTH WEEK'S EXERCISES.

Lie down and relax for a few minutes. Then sit up over your right side; stand up slowly and let's start with the Warm-up Exercises.

WARM-UPS.

1.	Arm Swinging.	10 X
2.	Knee Raising.	10 X
3.	Side Bend.	3 X
4.	Arm Circles.	10 X
5.	Shoulders Rolling.	5 X
6.	Squatting Down.	4 X
7.	Stretching Up.	2 X

SEVENTH WEEK'S YOGA EXERCISES.

BALANCING EXERCISE NO. 5 (Dancer's Pose). 1 version.

1. Stand on your right foot.
2. Raise your left foot up and reach for your toes with your left hand.
3. Stretch your right arm straight up.
4. Slowly bring your right arm forward and raise your left leg up.
5. Concentrate on one spot about 3-4 feet in front of you.
6. Hold for a few seconds.
7. Slowly lower your arm and leg down.

Repeat on left foot.

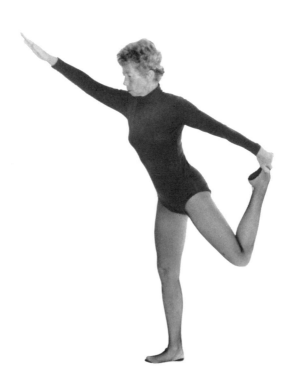

7TH WEEK.

WIDE KNEE BEND AND SHIFT.

1. Put your feet wider apart, than is comfortable.
2. Keep your feet parallel, toes pointing straight ahead.
3. Bend your right knee, keep left leg stretched.
4. Come up, shift over and bend left knee.

> 10 X count right knee

1. Stay down and shift from side to side.

> 10 X count right knee.

Try to go down a little bit deeper each time you practice and also do it more slowly. Feel how it works on your upper legs.

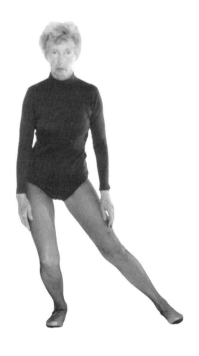

TRIANGLE POSTURE.

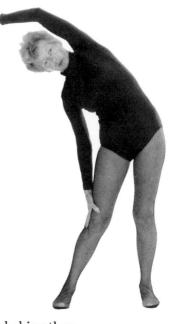

1. Put your feet comfortably apart.
2. Raise your arms, palms up, to shoulder height, while inhaling.
3. Turn your right hand around, bend down to your right side — exhale. Hold the position, do a gentle abdominal breathing.
4. Slowly raise your body up, turn your hands around while inhaling.
5. Bend down to your left side — exhale.
   Hold the position about 5 seconds, do a gentle abdominal breathing.
6. Slowly raise your body up.

Relax your legs by gently shaking them.

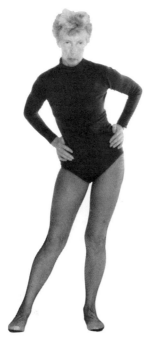

HIPROLLS.

1. Put your feet comfortably apart.
2. Put your hands on your hips.
3. Roll your hips gently around.

   10 X in each direction.

7TH WEEK.

PREPARATIONS FOR THE SUN EXERCISE.

UPPER LEG STRETCH.

1. Kneel down, put your hands in front of you.
2. Put your right foot forward between your hands.
3. Put your whole weight on your right foot, bring your knee forward.
4. Stretch your left leg back, resting on knee.
5. Put your fingertips down beside your foot.
6. Raise your head gently — inhale.
7. Put your head down — exhale.
8. Bring your right knee back to your left knee, relax your legs.

Repeat with your left leg.

HAMSTRING STRETCH.

1. Kneel down, put your hands in front of you.
2. Curl in your toes and stretch your legs.
3. Keep feet and hands where they are.
4. Gently and carefully bring your heels down a little.
5. Kneel down and relax your legs.

2 X

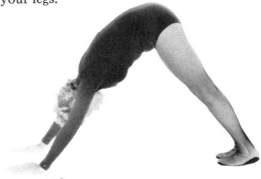

7TH WEEK.

PREPARATION FOR SUN EXERCISE.

THE STEP FORWARD.

1. Kneel down, put your hands in front of you.
2. Curl in your toes and stretch your legs.
3. Bring your right foot forward between your hands.
4. Stretch your right knee forward, your left leg back resting on knee.
5. Bring your right knee back to your left knee, relax your legs.

Repeat with left foot forward.

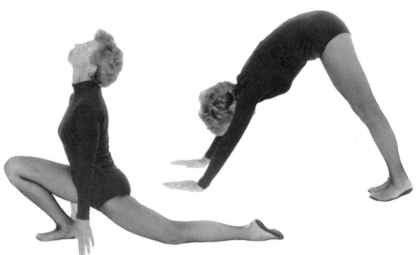

NOTE FOR TEACHERS.

Now is the time to demonstrate and explain the Sun Exercise, also called "The Salutation to the Sun." It is a sequence of twelve positions, which are done slowly one after the other in a smooth gentle way. They work through the whole body, especially bending the spine in every direction, and work on every muscle and connective tissue in the body. They also increase the blood circulation throughout the body. But even when you get warm doing this sequence, it is not a Warm-up because it starts with a stretch. You need gentle Warm-up exercises before you do the Sun. We have to practice one more position for it. Then we will put the whole sequence together.

180

7TH WEEK.

PREPARATION FOR SUN EXERCISE.

THE 8-POINT TOUCH.

1. Kneel down, put your hands in front of you.
2. Put your left foot forward between your hands.
3. Stretch your right leg back.
4. Now lift your right knee off the mat and bring your left foot back to your right foot (straight push-up position).
5. Put your knees down, keep feet on the mat.
6. Bend your arms, lower your chest down and your chin (now you know why we practiced push-ups). Your hips should be just about 5 inches off the floor to get a special bend in your lower back.

Lie down and r e l a x.

Repeat it once more after a short rest.

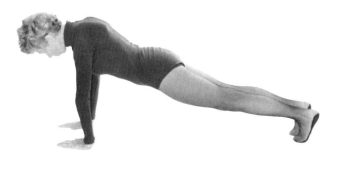

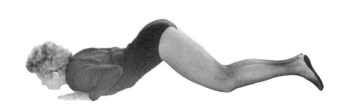

7TH WEEK.

In this exercise it is important to keep the body straight before you touch down, so that you automatically come to the right position. But the moment you bring your buttocks even a little bit out before going down, your hips will be too high and the position is hard to execute.

The Yoga exercises were originally created for men, by men, because 4000 years ago women did not go out of the house in India. Therefore many of the Yoga exercises have to be modified for women. This 8-point touch proves again that Yoga exercises were created for men. For women it should be named "the 9 point touch."

Now we are going to put the whole Sun Exercise together. It is a very beautiful sequence and after practicing it a few weeks you will enjoy it very much. The Yogis in India greet the sun with this sequence every morning before they start their regular exercise routine. Every pose is named after one month of the year and since the year has twelve months, they perform this sequence 12 times. Special emphasis is put on the breathing rhythm.

In the beginning do the sequence very gently, especially the backarching. Just let your head drop back slightly until your back gets more flexible.

Read the instructions first, then look at the pictures and try it gently and easily. Later on after a few weeks, you can stretch more and more with each one of the postures. But always remember, the gentle relaxed Warm-up exercises first, otherwise with cold or stiff muscles you can easily strain a muscle with the second posture, the stretch up and slightly backarch.

Do it very gently if pregnant.

THE SALUTATION TO THE SUN (SUN EXERCISE).

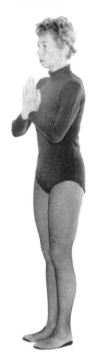

1. Put your hands together in front of your chest.

2. Raise your arms over your head while inhaling, bend your head back gently.

3. Bend forward while exhaling.

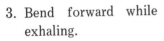

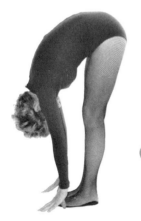

4. Put your hands down, stretch your right leg back, raise your head while inhaling.

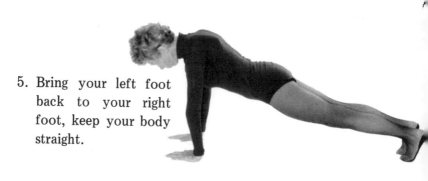

5. Bring your left foot back to your right foot, keep your body straight.

6. Put your knees down, lower your chest and your chin, exhale.

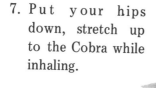

7. Put your hips down, stretch up to the Cobra while inhaling.

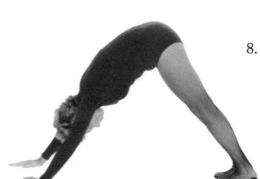

8. Curl in your toes, stretch up your hips while exhaling.

9. Bring your right foot forward between your hands, raise your head while inhaling.

10. Put your feet together in front, bend down while exhaling.

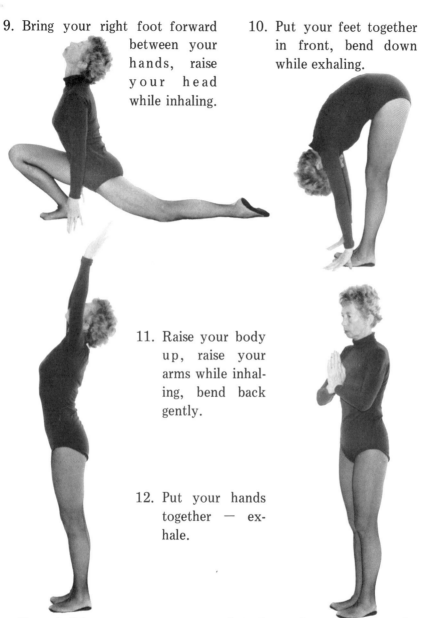

11. Raise your body up, raise your arms while inhaling, bend back gently.

12. Put your hands together — exhale.

Repeat this sequence once more, but change legs, that means in position 4 you stretch your left leg back, in position 9 you bring your left foot forward.

Lie down and r e l a x.

7TH WEEK.

THE BREATHING EXERCISES.

THE ABDOMINAL BREATHING.

1. Sit in cross-legged position, put your hands on your tummy.
2. Draw your tummy in — exhale.
3. Let your tummy go out — inhale.
4. Draw your tummy in — exhale.

5 X

THE MIDDLE OR RIBCAGE BREATHING.

1. Sit cross-legged, put your hands on your ribcage.
2. Squeeze your ribs gently together — exhale.
3. Expand your ribcage — inhale.
4. Feel your ribcage moving together — exhale.

5 X

THE UPPER OR CHEST BREATHING.

1. Sit cross-legged, put your fingertips on your collarbones.
2. Exhale, feel your chest going down.
3. Inhale slowly, feel your chest raising, your shoulders expanding.
4. Exhale, feel your chest going down.

5 X

Stretch your legs, relax your legs.

7TH WEEK.

FOOT EXERCISES.

1. In the sitting position put your hands behind you.
2. Stretch your feet, but don't point your toes, stretch your instep.
3. Stretch your heels, feel a gentle stretch in back of your calves.

5 X

1. Spread your legs slightly apart.
2. Roll your feet around in gentle circles.
3. Roll them in the opposite directions slowly and relaxed.

5 X

1. Raise your right leg slightly and shake it — put it down.
2. Raise your left leg slightly and shake it — put it down.
3. Raise both legs slightly and shake them — put them down.

Relax your legs.

THE COMPLETE BREATH.

Sit cross-legged or on a chair.
1. Draw your tummy in — exhale.
2. Let your tummy go out, expand your ribs and raise your chest while inhaling to the count of 8.
3. Draw your tummy in, your ribs go together, your chest goes down while exhaling to the count of 8.
4. There is three counts of rest, then inhale again.

5 X

THE LEG RAISING.

1. Lie completely relaxed, arms alongside your body.
2. Raise your right leg slowly while inhaling, gently stretch your heel.
3. Lower your right leg slowly while exhaling, keep your heel stretched going down.
4. Raise your left leg slowly while inhaling, gently stretch your heel.
5. Lower your left leg slowly while exhaling, keep your heel stretched going down.

2 X

1. Put your hands under your buttocks, palms down.
2. Raise both legs slowly while inhaling, gently stretch your heels.
3. Lower both legs slowly while exhaling, keep your heels stretched going down.

   Not for pregnant women.

2 X

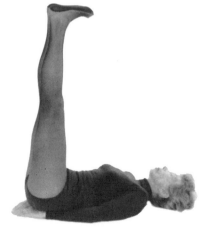

KNEE AND HEAD RAISING.

1. Raise your arms over your head while inhaling — s t r e t c h.
2. Bring your right knee up to your chest, put your hands and your head to your knee — exhale.
3. Put your head down, stretch your leg down, your arms up — inhale — s t r e t c h.
4. Bring your left knee up to your chest, put your hands and your head to your knee — exhale.
5. Put your head down, stretch your leg down, your arms up — inhale — s t r e t c h.
6. Bring both knees up to your chest, your hands to your knees, press them down — exhale.
7. Hold this position relaxed, relieve the pressure on your knees, but keep your hands around them. Relax your back, relax your arms, relax your shoulders.
8. Put your feet down first, then stretch your legs down, your arms up — inhale — s t r e t c h.
9. Bring your arms down — exhale and r e l a x.

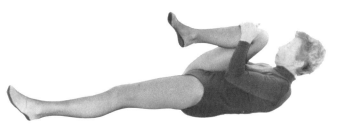

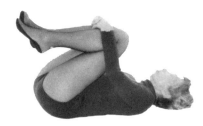

7TH WEEK.

WALK ON CEILING.

Another exercise again to strengthen different muscles in your abdominal area and your back.

1. Lie on your back, bring your knees high up to your chest.
2. Stretch your legs straight up and stretch your arms up.
3. Keep your legs stretched and move them about 2 feet forward and backward, the same with your arms. *Not for pregnant women*

About 10 X count right leg.

Watch the muscles in your back carefully, if you feel the slightest strain or discomfort, stop.

R e l a x.

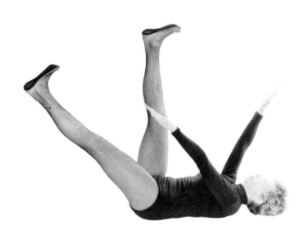

7TH WEEK.

NECK RELAXING MOVEMENTS.

1. Sit cross-legged or on chair.
2. Slowly let your head go down, chin toward chest.
3. Slowly raise your head up and bring it back.

5 X

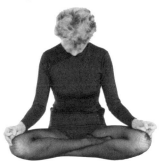 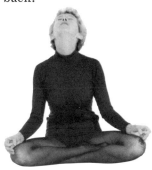

1. Slowly turn your head to your right side.
2. Slowly turn your head to your left side.

5 X

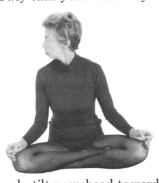 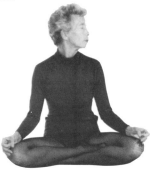

1. Slowly tilt your head toward your right shoulder.
2. Raise it up and tilt it slowly toward your left shoulder.

5 X

Stretch your legs and
relax your legs.

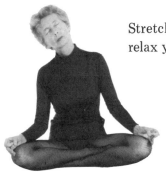 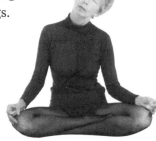

191

7TH WEEK.

ROCK AND ROLL.

1. Sit up, bend your knees, feet on mat.
2. Clasp your hands gently together under your knees.
3. Put your chin to your chest.
4. Swing your legs up gently and roll back to your shoulderblades.
5. Swing your legs down and roll up to your feet.

10 X

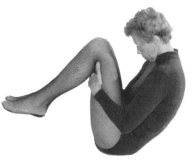 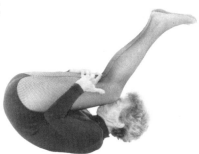

CROSS-LEGGED ROCK AND ROLL.

1. Sit up, cross your legs, hold on to your feet from the outside.
2. Lean back slightly, raise your feet about 10 inches off the mat.
3. Stretch your arms, so your feet get away from your body.
4. Slowly let yourself roll back, keep your knees bent.
5. Bring your feet fairly fast toward the crotch.
6. Let yourself roll up again.

5 X

Lie down and relax.

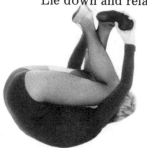 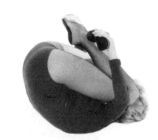

THE HALF SHOULDERSTAND.

1. Lie on your back, put your hands under your buttocks, starting with palms down.
2. Slowly raise your legs and hips, carry the weight of your hips on your hands.
3. Hold this position as long as you can easily and relaxed. Do a gentle abdominal breathing.
4. Lower your feet slightly farther over your head.
5. Put your hands on the mat, close together.
6. Bend your knees and slowly roll your back down, bring your hips down and stretch your legs down.

   R e l a x.

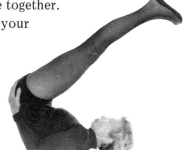

BACK RELAXING EXERCISES.

1. Lie on your back, bring your knees high up to your chest.
2. Put your hands on your knees, fingertips pointing toward your feet.
3. Slowly bring your knees closer to your chest.
4. Then slightly to your right side.
5. As far away from your chest as your arms can reach.
6. Slightly to your left side.
7. And to your chest again. Repeat these gentle circles 5 X in each direction.

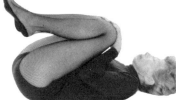

193

7TH WEEK.

KNEE TO FOREHEAD POSE. (Preparation for Plow Posture.)

We go first into the Half Shoulderstand.

1. Lie on your back, put your hands under your buttocks, starting with palms down.
2. Slowly raise your legs and hips.
3. Bring your legs slowly farther over your head, as far as you can without feeling any strain in your neck, back or head.
4. Bend your knees and put them on your forehead.
5. Hold for a few seconds.
6. Put your hands on the mat, keep your knees bent and slowly roll your back down and stretch your legs down.

2 X

Lie down and relax.

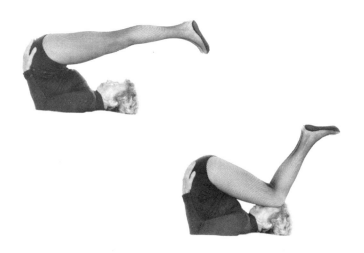

7TH WEEK.

SIT UP AND ROLL DOWN.

To strengthen your abdominal muscles and to relax your back and neck muscles.

1. Lie on your back, bend your knees slightly, feet flat on mat.
2. Raise your arms over your head.
3. Swing your arms up, roll your body up, bend forward relaxed.
4. Keep your arms beside your body and slowly roll your back down, keep your chin to your chest to the last moment. Feel every vertebrae rolling down.

3 X

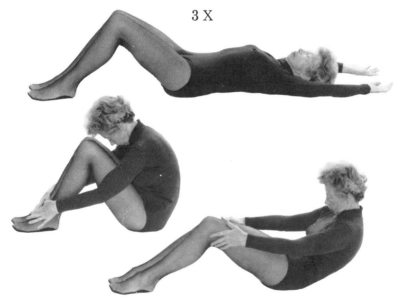

If you have trouble coming up, then roll on your side and come up over your right side. The important part of this exercise is the rolling down. During this slow rolling down movement your abdominal muscles get strengthened and it also will firm up your tummy, which the sit-up movement does not do.

After a few weeks you will also be able to come up more easily, without straining, but always concentrate on the rolling down part and do it more slowly every time.

It works also on relaxing your back muscles and makes you ready for the next more advanced exercise.

7TH WEEK.

STRAIGHT SHOULDERSTAND. (Candle Posture.)

Strengthens the neck, shoulder and upper back muscles. Makes the neck more flexible. Increases the blood circulation in the thyroid glands.

1. Lie on your back, put your hands under your buttocks, starting with palms down.
2. Slowly raise your legs and your hips, support your hips with your hands. (Half Shoulderstand).
3. Now very slowly stretch your legs straighter up and slide your hands to your back, support yourself well, elbows on the mat.
4. To come down; *first lower your hips down,* slide your hands to your hips, at the same time your legs are coming down over your face and you are in the Half Shoulderstand again.
5. Bring your legs farther over your head, put your hands down on the mat, close together, bend your knees and slowly roll your body down. Bring your legs down and *r e l a x.*

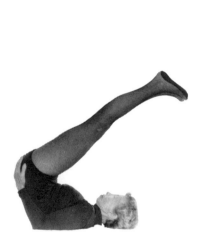 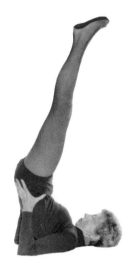

Even if you are not able to stretch up completely straight in the beginning, you will get the benefits of this posture already. If your chin is pressing slightly against your chest, the blood circulation in your thyroid glands is increased. So don't work too hard on it. Especially watch it in the morning.

If you feel that the straight Shoulderstand is just a little bit too much for you, then don't do it yet. Keep practicing all the other exercises. Your abdominal and back muscles need some more work to get the strength to hold your body up or also to bring it up into the position. Also if you did feel kind of wiggly, wait just a few more weeks and then try it again.

Through stretching the body up, the chin is pressed against the chest. This is called the chin lock. By means of the chin lock, the blood circulation to the head is slightly decreased and the blood circulation in the neck is increased. The thyroid glands are located in the front of the neck, so with this position the blood circulation in the thyroid glands is increased. This can bring the thyroid glands back to better working order. It will *regulate* the work of these glands. The thyroid glands control your weight, so if you are overweight you will loose some pounds, or if you are underweight you will gain. Through practicing Yoga you will, in time, get the perfect weight for your body build.

When practicing the Shoulderstand be careful in the beginning. Always go very slowly into the position and work very slowly up to longer holding times. Come down very slowly and rest for a few minutes so the blood circulation goes slowly back to normal again.

7TH WEEK.

BRIDGE POSTURE.

1. Lie on your back, arms relaxed alongside your body.
2. Bend your knees, put your feet on the mat slightly apart.
3. Slowly raise your hips while inhaling.
4. Lower your hips while exhaling, press your back down, draw your tummy in.

3 X

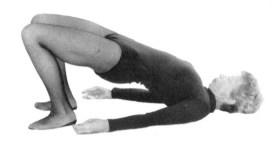

CRAWLING.

1. Get on your hands and knees.
2. Bring your right knee and your left hand forward.
3. Bring your left knee and your right hand forward. Keep doing this and crawl around your living room in big circles.

    If you feel comfortable increase it now to 3 rounds. But watch your body, especially your arm and shoulder muscles.

Lie down and r e l a x.

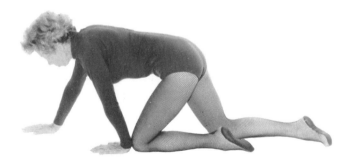

THE RELAXING POSTURE.

Close your eyes and lie in the most comfortable position. Arms slightly away from your body. Palms turned up. Shoulders relaxed.

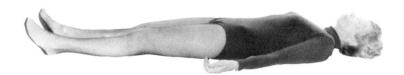

Relax your legs.
Relax your feet.
Relax your toes.
Relax your calves.
Relax your thighs.
Relax your stomach.
Relax your chest.
Relax your shoulders.
Relax your arms.
Relax your hands.
Relax your fingers.
Relax your neck.
Relax your head.
Relax your face.
Relax your mouth.
Relax your teeth.
Relax every muscle in your back.
Relax your whole body.
Relax completely.

Relax for about 10 minutes. Then raise your arms over your head and s t r e t c h, roll on your left side and s t r e t c h, roll on your right side and s t r e t c h. Sit up over your right side.

Thank you, see you tomorrow.

7TH WEEK.

SUMMARY

SEVENTH WEEK'S EXERCISES.

WARM-UPS.

1.	Arm Swinging.	10 X
2.	Knee Raising.	10 X
3.	Side Bend.	3 X each side.
4.	Arm Circles.	10 X
5.	Shoulders Rolling.	5 X
6.	Squatting Down.	4 X
7.	Stretching Up.	2 X

YOGA EXERCISES.

1. Balancing Exercise No. 5. (Dancer's Pose. 1. Version.) 1 X each foot.
2. Wide Knee Bend and Shift. 10 X
3. Triangle. 5 seconds.
4. Hiprolls. 10 X each direction.
5. Upper Leg Stretch. 1 X each leg.
6. Hamstring Stretch. 2 X
7. The Step Forward. 1 X each foot.
8. *The 8-Point Touch.* 2 X
9. *The Salutation to the Sun. (Sun Exercise.)* 2 X
10. The Breathing Exercises. 5 X each.
11. The Foot Exercises. 5 X each.
12. The Complete Breath. 5 X. Relax.
13. The Leg Raising. 2 X each.
14. Knee and Head Raising. 1 X each. Relax.
15. *Walk on Ceiling.* 10 X. Relax.
16. Neck Relaxing Movements. 5 X each.
17. Rock and Roll. 10 X
18. Cross-legged Rock and Roll. 5 X. Relax.
19. The Half Shoulderstand. Hold as long as comfortable.

20. Back Relaxing Exercise. 5 X each direction.
21. Knee to Forehead Pose. 2 X. Relax.
22. *Sit Up and Roll Down.* 3 X
23. *Straight Shoulderstand.* 2 X. Relax.
24. Bridge Posture. 3 X
25. Crawling. 3 rounds.
26. The Relaxing Posture.

EIGHTH WEEK'S EXERCISES.

Lie down and relax for a few minutes. Then sit up over your right side; stand up slowly and let's start with the Warm-Up exercises.

WARM-UPS.

1.	Arm Swinging.	10 X
2.	Knee Raising.	10 X
3.	Side Bend.	3 X
4.	Arm Circles.	10 X
5.	Shoulders Rolling.	5 X
6.	Squatting Down.	4 X
7.	Stretching Up.	2 X

EIGHTH WEEK'S YOGA EXERCISES.

BALANCING EXERCISE NO. 6. (Dancer's Pose.) 2. Version.

1. Stand on your right foot.
2. Raise your left foot up and reach for your toes with your left hand.
3. Stretch your right arm straight up.
4. Slowly bring your right arm forward and raise your left leg up.
5. Concentrate on one spot about 3-4 feet in front of you.
6. Now slowly bring your leg higher up and stretch your arm straight up. Feel the gentle stretch in your back and your upper leg.
7. Slowly lower your arm and leg down.

Repeat on left foot.

Not for pregnant women.

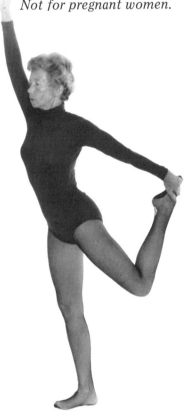

203

8TH WEEK.

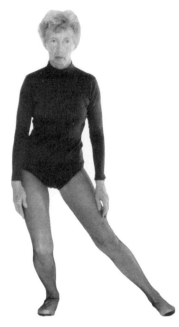

WIDE KNEE BEND AND SHIFT.

1. Put your feet wider apart than is comfortable.
2. Keep your feet parallel, toes pointing straight ahead.
3. Bend your right knee, keep left leg stretched.
4. Come up, shift over and bend left knee.

10 X

1. Stay down and shift from side to side.

10 X

TRIANGLE POSTURE.

1. Put your feet comfortably apart.
2. Raise your arms, palms up to shoulder height, while inhaling.
3. Turn your right hand around, bend down to your right side — exhale. Hold the position, do a gentle abdominal breathing. 5 seconds.
4. Slowly raise your body up, turn your hands around — inhale.
5. Bend down to your left side — exhale.
   Hold the position, do a gentle abdominal breathing. 5 seconds.
6. Slowly raise your body up.

Relax your legs by gently shaking them.

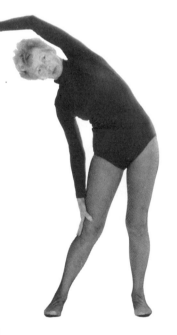

8TH WEEK.

HIPROLLS.

1. Put your feet comfortably apart.
2. Put your hands on your hips.
3. Roll your hips around gently.

    10 X in each direction.

ARMSTRETCH.

1. Put your feet comfortably apart.
2. Fold your hands behind your back, just fingertips crossing.
3. Raise your arms behind your back as high as you can without feeling any strain, keep your body straight.
4. Bend forward completely relaxed, keep raising your arms.
5. Slowly raise your body up, your arms are coming down.
    Relax your arms, relax your shoulders.

    2 X

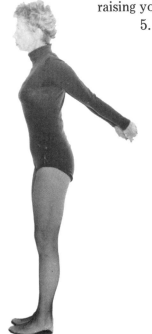

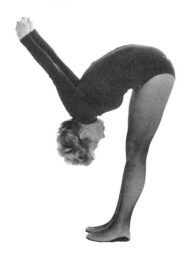

ARMSTRETCH VARIATION.

1. Put your right foot forward one step; turn your left foot 45°.
2. Bend your left knee, fold your hands behind your back.
3. Raise your arms behind your back, bend slowly forward over your right leg.
4. Slowly raise your body up, relax your legs.

Repeat with left leg in front.

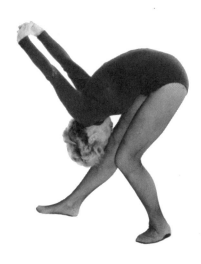

THE SALUTATION TO THE SUN. (SUN EXERCISE.)

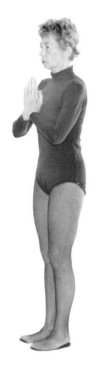

1. Put your hands together in front of your chest.

2. Raise your arms over your head while inhaling, bend your head back gently.

3. Bend forward while exhaling.

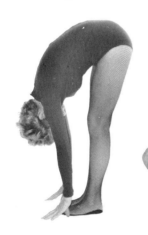

4. Put your hands down, stretch your right leg back, raise your head while inhaling.

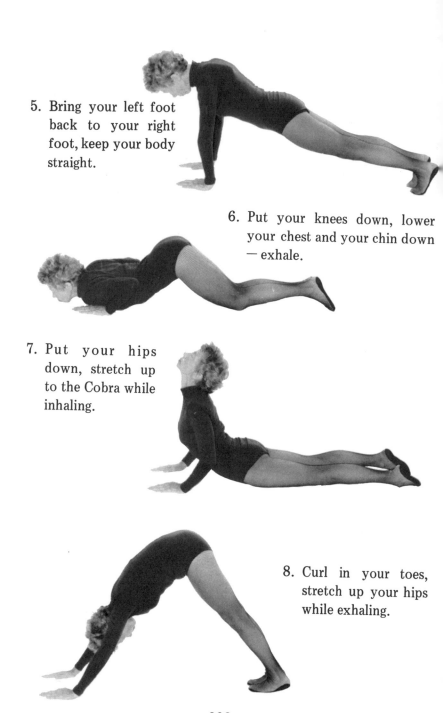

5. Bring your left foot back to your right foot, keep your body straight.

6. Put your knees down, lower your chest and your chin down — exhale.

7. Put your hips down, stretch up to the Cobra while inhaling.

8. Curl in your toes, stretch up your hips while exhaling.

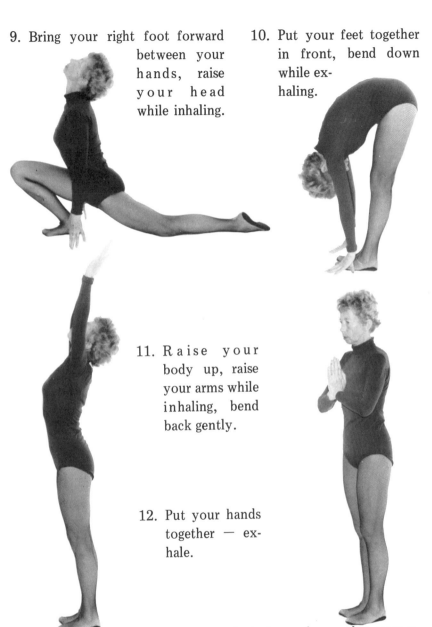

9. Bring your right foot forward between your hands, raise your head while inhaling.

10. Put your feet together in front, bend down while exhaling.

11. Raise your body up, raise your arms while inhaling, bend back gently.

12. Put your hands together — exhale.

Repeat this sequence once more, but change legs — that means:
In position 4 you stretch your left leg back,
in position 9 you bring your left foot forward.

Lie down and r e l a x.

THE BREATHING EXERCISES.

THE ABDOMINAL BREATHING.

1. Sit in cross-legged position, put your hands on your tummy.
2. Draw your tummy in — exhale.
3. Let your tummy go out — inhale.
4. Draw your tummy in — exhale.

5 X

THE MIDDLE OR RIBCAGE BREATHING.

1. Sit cross-legged, put your hands on your ribcage.
2. Squeeze your ribs gently together — exhale.
3. Expand your ribcage — inhale.
4. Feel your ribs moving together — exhale.

5 X

THE UPPER OR CHEST BREATHING.

1. Sit cross-legged, put your fingertips on your collarbones.
2. Exhale, feel your chest going down.
3. Inhale, feel your chest raising, your shoulders expanding.
4. Exhale, feel your chest going down.

5 X

Stretch your legs, relax your legs by gently shaking them.

8TH WEEK.

FOOT EXERCISES.

1. In the sitting position put your hands behind you.
2. Stretch your feet, but don't point your toes, stretch your instep.
3. Stretch your heels, feel a gentle stretch in back of your calves.

5 X

1. Spread your legs slightly apart.
2. Roll your feet around in gentle circles.
3. Roll them in the opposite directions slowly and relaxed.

5 X

1. Raise your right leg slightly and shake it — put it down.
2. Raise your left leg slightly and shake it — put it down.
3. Raise both legs slightly and shake them — put them down.

Relax your legs.

THE COMPLETE BREATH.

After several weeks of practicing the Complete Breath you know the technique well. Now try to concentrate during breathing on the energy you take in with the oxygen. It is called Prana, the life force. You take it in with your breath. It stays in your body, only the carbon dioxide goes out again. Feel it going into every cell of your body. Find fresh air and breathe the energy into your lungs and your cells.

Sit cross-legged or on a chair.
1. Draw your tummy in — exhale.
2. Let your tummy go out, expand your ribs, raise your chest while inhaling to the count of 8.
3. Draw your tummy in, your ribs go together, your chest goes down while exhaling to the count of 8.
4. There is three counts of rest.

5 X

211

THE LEG RAISING.

1. Lie completely relaxed, arms alongside your body.
2. Raise your right leg slowly while inhaling, gently stretch your heel.
3. Lower your right leg while exhaling, keep your heel stretched going down.
4. Raise your left leg slowly while inhaling, gently stretch your heel.
5. Lower your left leg slowly while exhaling, keep your heel stretched going down.

2 X

1. Put your hands under your buttocks, palms down.
2. Raise both legs slowly while inhaling, gently stretch your heels.
3. Lower both legs slowly while exhaling, keep your heels stretched going down.

Not for pregnant women.

2 X

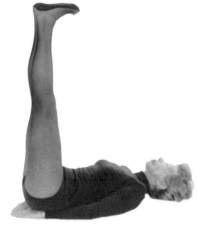

8TH WEEK.

KNEE AND HEAD RAISING.

1. Raise your arms over your head while inhaling — stretch.
2. Bring your right knee up to your chest, put your hands and your head to your knee — exhale.
3. Put your head down, stretch your leg down, your arms up — inhale — stretch.
4. Bring your left knee up to your chest, put your hands and your head to your knee — exhale.
5. Put your head down, stretch your leg down, your arms up — inhale.
6. Bring both knees up to your chest, your hands to your knees, press them down — exhale.
7. Hold the position relaxed, relieve the pressure on your knees, but keep your hands around them. Relax your back, relax your arms, relax your shoulders.
8. Put your feet down first, then stretch your legs down, your arms up — inhale — stretch.
9. Bring your arms down — exhale and relax.

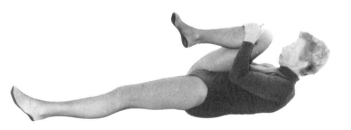

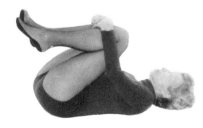

8TH WEEK.

LEG OVER.

To stretch and strengthen the lateral stomach muscles.
To slim down hips, buttocks and upper legs.

1. Stretch your arms out to the sides.
2. Raise your right leg slowly straight up.
3. Bring it slowly over in direction toward your left hand.
4. Slowly raise it up and put it down.
   Repeat with your left leg.

2 X

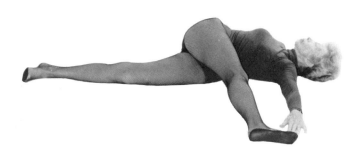

NECK RELAXING MOVEMENTS.

1. Sit cross-legged or on chair.
2. Slowly let your head go down, chin to chest.
3. Slowly raise your head up and bring it back.

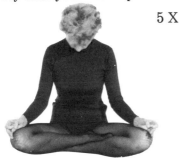

5 X

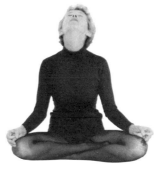

1. Slowly turn your head to your right side.
2. Slowly turn your head to your left side.

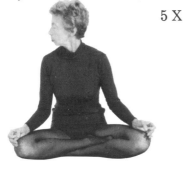

5 X

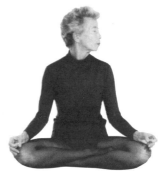

1. Slowly tilt your head toward your right shoulder.
2. Raise it up and tilt it slowly toward your left shoulder.

5 X

Stretch your legs,
relax your legs.
Lie down and relax.

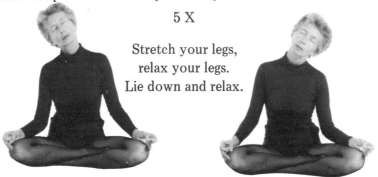

8TH WEEK.

ROCK AND ROLL.

1. Sit up, bend your knees, feet on mat.
2. Clasp your hands gently together under your knees.
3. Put your chin to your chest.
4. Swing your legs up gently and roll back to your shoulderblades.
5. Swing your legs down and roll up to your feet.

10 X

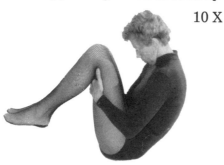
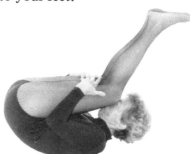

CROSS-LEGGED ROCK AND ROLL.

1. Sit up, cross your legs, hold on to your feet from the outside.
2. Lean back slightly, raise your feet about 10 inches off the mat.
3. Stretch your arms, so your feet get away from your body.
4. Slowly let yourself roll back, keep your knees bent.
5. Bring your feet fairly fast toward the crotch.
6. Let yourself roll up again.

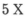

5 X

Lie down and relax.

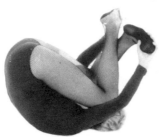
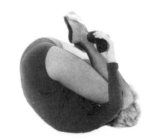

216

THE HALF SHOULDERSTAND WITH BALANCE.

Gives the same benefits as the normal Half Shoulderstand.
Relieves strain on back.

1. Lie on your back, put your hands under your buttocks, starting with palms down.
2. Slowly raise your legs and hips; carry the weight of your hips on your hands.
3. Now raise your hips just a little bit higher and try to lift your elbows off the mat.
4. When you feel you can balance in this position, then slide your hands up your legs and hold with stretched arms on to your legs, wherever you can reach.
5. Slide your hands down to your hips, bring your feet slightly farther over your head.
6. Put your hands on the mat, close together.
7. Bend your knees and slowly roll your back down, bring your hips down and stretch your legs down.

   2 X

Watch it that your feet are still higher than your hips, so you get the benefits of the slanting position of your legs. Some people have difficulties balancing in this position at first. It takes some practice. But it also depends on the body build.

Even after trying it several times, some people just cannot do it. Don't worry about it, just practice the Half Shoulderstand with your elbows on the mat. You will get more benefits if you can hold this one relaxed and with ease than from trying too hard to hold your balance with your arms up on your legs.

BACK RELAXING EXERCISE.

1. Lie on your back, bring your knees high up to your chest.
2. Put your hands on your knees, fingertips pointing toward your feet.
3. Slowly make circles with your knees. Bring them very close to your chest, slightly to your right side, far away from your chest, slightly to your left side.

5 X in each direction.

Feel the relaxing effect on your back muscles.

Stretch your legs and relax.

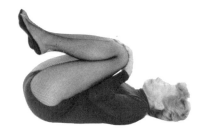

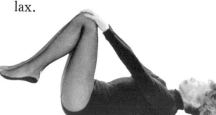

KNEE TO FOREHEAD POSE.

1. Lie on your back, put your hands under your buttocks, starting with palms down.
2. Slowly raise your legs and your hips.
3. Bring your legs slowly farther over your head as far as you can without feeling any strain in your back, neck or head.
4. Bend your knees and put them on your forehead.
5. Hold for 5-10 seconds.
6. Put your hands on the mat, keep your knees bent and slowly roll your back down, bring your hips down and stretch your legs down.

2 X

Lie down and relax.

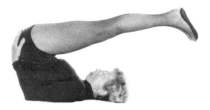

PLOW POSTURE AND KNEE TO EAR POSE.

Makes the spine more flexible.

Increases blood circulation in the abdominal organs.

Massages the intestines, increases peristaltic movement, relieves constipation.

Slims down and firms up hips, buttocks and tummy.

1. Lie on your back, put your hands under your buttocks, starting with palms down.
2. Slowly raise your legs and hips.
3. Bring your legs slowly farther over your head. Watch your back, neck and head. (You should not feel any strain. If you do, you are going too far for the flexibility of your back and neck muscles.) If you can touch your toes to the mat over your head, you accomplished the Plow Posture.
4. Hold it for a few seconds.
5. Then bend your knees and put them on your forehead or put them down beside your ears to the Knee to Ear Pose. (But don't force them down.)
6. Put your hands on the mat, keep your knees bent and slowly roll your back down, bring your hips down and stretch your legs down.

2 X

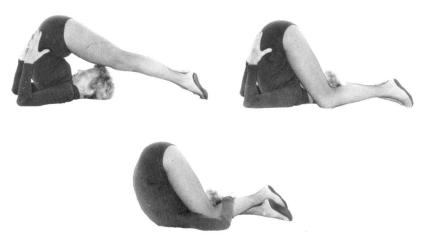

219

Caution: Only touch your toes to the mat for the Plow Posture if you don't feel any strain in your back, neck or your head. Also you should not feel any pressure in your head. If you should get a choking feeling while trying to do the Plow Posture, then your body is not prepared enough for this posture. So take your time and be patient. One day you will be able to do it easily and relaxed. But always before doing it, limber up your neck and back with the *Neck Movements, followed by the Rock and Roll, followed by the Half Shoulderstand. Then you can try the Plow Posture.* One more point which is important. Some people just cannot do the Plow Posture because of their body build. Any person with a long upper body will have problems with it. These people should do the Knee to Forehead Pose and will get the same benefits. Also watch your hamstrings. The connective tissue there is very tight and it takes a long time to stretch.

BRIDGE POSTURE.

1. Lie on your back, arms relaxed alongside your body.
2. Bend your knees, put your feet on the mat closely to your body and slightly apart.
3. Slowly raise your hips while inhaling.
4. Lower your hips while exhaling, press your back down, draw your tummy in.

3 X

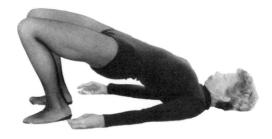

Lie down and relax.

FORWARD BEND.

1. Sit up slowly over your right side and spread your legs apart.
2. Slowly raise your arms at your sides over your head while inhaling.
3. Put your hands on your right knee or leg, bend down while exhaling.
4. Slide your hands up your leg, raise your arms at your sides over your head while inhaling.
5. Bend down over your left leg while exhaling.

2 X

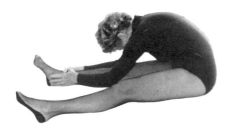

1. Bring your legs together, raise your arms at your sides while inhaling.
2. Bend down over both legs while exhaling.

2 X

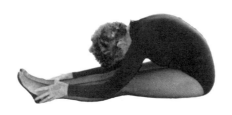

Relax your legs by shaking them gently.

221

THE ALTERNATE LEG BEND.

1. In the sitting position spread your legs apart.
2. Put the sole of your left foot against the inside of your right thigh.
3. Raise your arms at your sides over your head while inhaling.
4. Bend slowly down over your stretched leg while exhaling.

2 X

Stretch your leg, relax your legs.

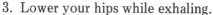

1. Spread your legs apart again.
2. Put the sole of your right foot against the inside of your left thigh.
3. Raise your arms at your sides over your head while inhaling.
4. Bend slowly down over your stretched leg while exhaling.

2 X

Stretch your leg, relax your legs.
Lie down and relax.

THE PLANE.

1. In the sitting position put your hands behind you.
2. Slowly raise your hips while inhaling, stretch your whole body, let your head go back.
3. Lower your hips while exhaling.

2 X

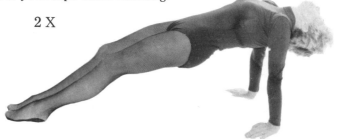

Relax your wrists, relax your arms, relax your legs by gently shaking them.

Lie down and relax.

8TH WEEK.

SPINAL TWIST. (THIRD VERSION.)

1. Sit up slowly, spread your legs slightly apart.
2. Put your right foot under your left thigh.
3. Put your left foot over your right knee.
4. Put your right hand on your left foot.
5. Stretch your left arm forward, keep looking at your hand and slowly bring your left arm back, then bend it and put it around your back, keep looking over your left shoulder.
6. Stretch your arm and bring it slowly forward looking at your hand.
7. Put your arm down, stretch your leg, relax your legs.

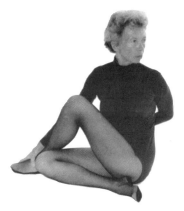

Now the other side.

1. Sit up straight, spread your legs slightly apart.
2. Put your left foot under your right thigh.
3. Put your right foot over your left knee.
4. Put your left hand on your right foot.
5. Stretch your right arm forward, keep looking at your hand and slowly bring your right arm back, then bend it and put it around your back, keep looking over your right shoulder.
6. Stretch your arm and bring it slowly forward looking at your hand.
7. Put your arm down, stretch your leg, relax your legs.

Lie down and relax.

CAT STRETCH NO. 1.

To relax the muscles in your back.

1. Sit up slowly and get on your hands and knees.
2. Slowly bring your right knee toward your forehead, make your back round.
3. Slowly stretch your right leg back and raise your head up.

5 X with each leg.

Put your feet over to one side, sit down on the other side, stretch your legs, relax your legs and lie down and relax.

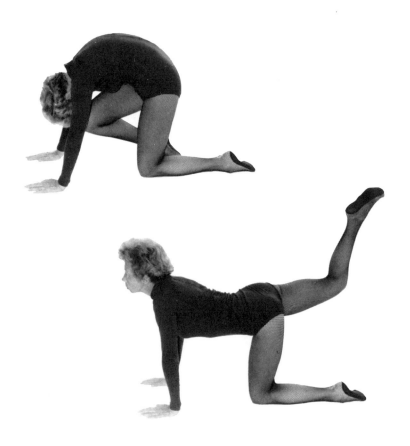

CRAWLING.

1. Get on your hands and knees.
2. Bring your right knee and your left hand forward.
3. Bring your left knee and your right hand forward.

   Keep doing that and crawl around your living room in big circles. If you feel comfortable increase it to 3 rounds now. But watch your body, especially your arm and shoulder muscles.

   Lie down and r e l a x.

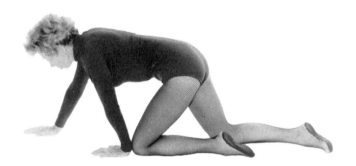

8TH WEEK.

THE RELAXING POSTURE.

Close your eyes and lie in the most comfortable position. Arms slightly away from your body. Palms up. Shoulders relaxed.

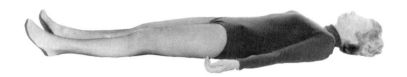

Relax your legs.
Relax your feet.
Relax your toes.
Relax your calves.
Relax your thighs.
Relax your stomach.
Relax your chest.
Relax your shoulders.
Relax your arms.
Relax your hands.
Relax your fingers.
Relax your neck.
Relax your head.
Relax your face.
Relax your mouth.
Relax your teeth.
Relax every muscle in your back.
Relax your whole body.
Relax completely.

Relax for 10 minutes. Then raise your arms over your head and s t r e t c h, roll on your left side and s t r e t c h, roll on your right side and s t r e t c h. Sit up over your right side.

Thank you, see you tomorrow.

8TH WEEK.

SUMMARY

EIGHTH WEEK'S EXERCISES.

WARM-UPS.

1. Arm Swinging.   10 X
2. Knee Raising.   10 X
3. Side Bend.   3 X each side.
4. Arm Circles.   10 X
5. Shoulders Rolling.   5 X
6. Squatting Down.   4 X
7. Stretching Up.   2 X

YOGA EXERCISES.

1. *Balancing Exercise No. 6.* (Dancer's Pose. 2. Version.)
   1 X each foot.
2. Wide Knee Bend and Shift. 10 X
3. Triangle. 5 seconds each side.
4. Hiprolls. 10 each direction.
5. Armstretch. 2 X
6. *Armstretch Variation.* 1 X each leg.
7. The Salutation to the Sun. 2 X
8. The 3 Parts of Breathing. 5 X each.
9. The Foot Exercises. About 5 X each.
10. The Complete Breath. 5 X
11. The Leg Raising. 2 X
12. Knee and Head Raising. 1 X each. Relax.
13. *Leg Over.* 2 X to each side. Relax.
14. Neck Relaxing Movements. 5 X each.
15. Rock and Roll. 10 X
16. Cross-legged Rock and Roll. 5 X. Relax.
17. *The Half Shoulderstand with Balance.* 2 X
18. Back Relaxing Exercise. 5 X in each direction.
19. Knee to Forehead Pose. 2 X. Relax.

20. *Plow Posture and Knee to Ear Pose.* 2 X. Relax.
21. Bridge Posture. 3 X. Relax.
22. Forward Bend. 2 X each.
23. The Alternate Leg Bend. 2 X
24. The Plane. 2 X. Relax.
25. *The Spinal Twist. 3. Version.* 1 X each side. Relax.
26. *Catstretch No. 1.* 5 X each leg.
27. Crawling. 3 rounds.
28. The Relaxing Posture.

NINTH WEEK'S EXERCISES.

Lie down and relax for a few minutes. Then sit up over your right side; stand up slowly and let's start with the Warm-up exercises.

WARM-UPS.

1.	Arm Swinging.	10 X
2.	Knee Raising.	10 X
3.	Side Bend.	3 X each side.
4.	Arm Circles.	10 X
5.	Shoulders Rolling.	5 X
6.	Squatting Down.	4 X
7.	Stretching Up.	2 X

Now your muscles are limbered up, the blood circulates well, the stiffness is out of your joints, so let's do the Sun Exercise.

9TH WEEK.

THE SALUTATION TO THE SUN. (SUN EXERCISE.)

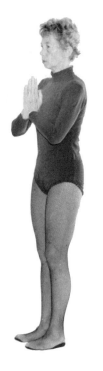

1. Put your hands together in front of your chest.

2. Raise your arms over your head while inhaling, bend your head back gently.

3. Bend forward while exhaling.

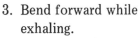

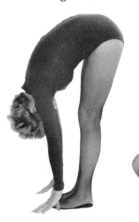

4. Put your hands down, stretch your right leg back, raise your head while inhaling.

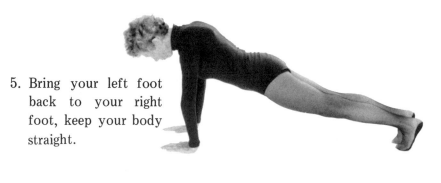

5. Bring your left foot back to your right foot, keep your body straight.

6. Put your knees down, lower your chest and your chin — exhale.

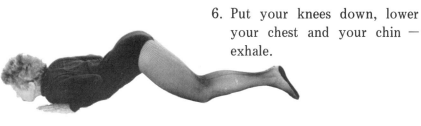

7. Put your hips down, stretch up to the Cobra while inhaling.

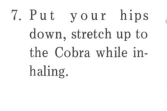

8. Curl in your toes, stretch up your hips while exhaling.

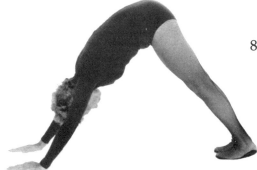

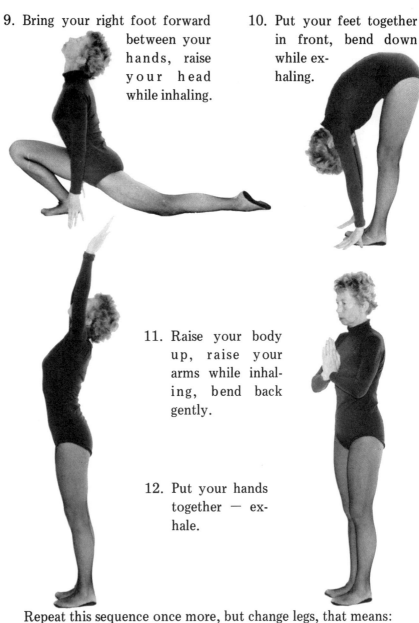

9. Bring your right foot forward between your hands, raise your head while inhaling.

10. Put your feet together in front, bend down while exhaling.

11. Raise your body up, raise your arms while inhaling, bend back gently.

12. Put your hands together — exhale.

Repeat this sequence once more, but change legs, that means:
In position 4 you stretch your left leg back,
in position 9 you bring your left foot forward.

Lie down and r e l a x.

Some people will have trouble with position No. 9 of the Sun Exercise. To bring the foot forward between the hands is not an easy step. Because of body build it is nearly impossible for some persons to execute it this way.

If you are not able to do it despite practicing it over and over again, kneel down first and then put the foot forward the same way we did when we practiced the preparations for the Sun Exercise.

The benefits of the Sun Exercise are so great, it would be a pity to give it up because of this one difficult movement.

The whole Sun Exercise is not an easy sequence; it is not for straight beginners. We have to work up to it slowly, to be able to enjoy it. The longer you practice this sequence the more you will enjoy it. When it starts to become easy, then stretch just a little bit more each time and breathe more deeply. The deeper you breathe the more slowly you will perform the sequence. Let every position flow gently into the next one.

After doing it for a few weeks regularly every day, try to perform it with your eyes closed and direct your consciousness to your spine.

THE BREATHING EXERCISES.

THE 3 PARTS OF BREATHING.

THE ABDOMINAL BREATHING.

1. Sit in cross-legged position, put your hands on your tummy.
2. Draw your tummy in — exhale.
3. Let your tummy go out — inhale.
4. Draw your tummy in — exhale.

5 X

THE MIDDLE OR RIBCAGE BREATHING.

1. Sit cross-legged, put your hands on your ribcage.
2. Squeeze your ribs gently together — exhale.
3. Expand your ribcage — inhale.
4. Feel your ribs moving together — exhale.

5 X

THE UPPER OR CHEST BREATHING.

1. Sit cross-legged, put your fingertips on your collarbones.
2. Exhale, feel your chest going down.
3. Inhale — feel your chest raising, your shoulders expanding.
4. Exhale, feel your chest going down.

5 X

Stretch your legs, relax your legs by gently shaking them.

9TH WEEK.

FOOT EXERCISES.

1. In the sitting position put your hands behind you.
2. Stretch your feet, but don't point your toes, stretch your instep.
3. Stretch your heels, feel a gentle stretch in back of your calves.

5 X

1. Spread your legs slightly apart.
2. Roll your feet around in gentle circles.
3. Roll them in the opposite directions slowly and relaxed.

5 X

1. Raise your right leg slightly and shake it — put it down.
2. Raise your left leg slightly and shake it — put it down.
3. Raise both legs slightly and shake them — put them down.

Relax your legs.

9TH WEEK.

THE COMPLETE BREATH WITH COLOR.

To become even more conscious of your breathing, we are going to breathe with color today. You try to picture the air you are inhaling your favorite color, perhaps light green. You close your eyes during inhalation and feel and see the beautiful light green fresh oxygen come into your lungs.

First if spreads out in the lower part of your lungs, then in the middle part and the upper part. It goes from the lungs into the bloodstream. And now the carbon dioxide with the toxins and waste products comes back to your lungs — it does not have the beautiful light green color any more — it is dark and dirty. Breathe it out of your lungs, see it coming out, first out of the lowest part of your lungs, then the middle part and then the upper part. Try to exhale even longer than you inhaled to get it out.

It will not be easy, it takes a lot of concentration, but by now you should be able to concentrate well enough to accomplish it.

1. Sit cross-legged or on a chair.
2. Draw your tummy in — exhale.
3. Let your tummy go out, expand your ribs, raise your chest while inhaling the beautiful light green fresh oxygen.
4. Draw your tummy in, your ribs go together, your chest goes down while exhaling the dark dirty carbon dioxide.

5 X

Lie down and relax.

After doing this breathing exercise with one of my classes, I asked about the reaction and the feelings they got; if it was easy, if they could concentrate on the color?

One student said: she could concentrate all right on the color, but she had a hard time finding light green fresh air after the first exhalation. She had the feeling there was a cloud of dark green dirty air sitting in front of her nose.

With this breathing exercise you will realize how important it is to live in well-ventilated, smoke free and airy rooms.

9TH WEEK.

THE LEG RAISING.

Our Leg Raising exercise now changes slightly. Your muscles and connective tissues are stretched enough to try gently the next move. After raising the leg we slide the hands up and bring the stretched leg closer toward the body to stretch the muscles and connective tissues just a little bit more. It also slims down buttocks and hips. But do it very carefully. You should not feel any strain, just a gentle stretch. You should never feel a burning sensation in the back of your upper leg. If you do, you are stretching too much.

This movement also prepares your legs for another more advanced posture.

1. Lie completely relaxed, arms alongside your body.
2. Inhale — raise your right leg slowly, slide your hands up your leg and bring it gently closer.
3. Lower your right leg while exhaling.
4. Inhale — raise your left leg slowly, slide your hands up your leg, bring it gently closer.
5. Lower your left leg slowly while exhaling.
   Do not bounce your leg.

2 X

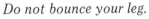

1. Put your hands under your buttocks, palms down.
2. Inhale — raise both legs slowly, slide your hands up your legs, bring them gently closer.
3. Put your hands under your buttocks again, lower your legs slowly while exhaling.

Not for pregnant women.

2 X

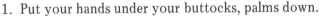

Don't raise your hips.

KNEE AND HEAD RAISING.

1. Raise your arms over your head while inhaling — stretch.
2. Bring your right knee up to your chest, put your hands and your head to your knee — exhale.
3. Put your head down, stretch your leg down, your arms up — inhale — stretch.
4. Bring your left knee up to your chest, your hands and your head to your knee — exhale.
5. Put your head down, stretch your leg down, your arms up — inhale — stretch.
6. Bring both knees up to your chest, your hands to your knees, press them down — exhale.
7. Hold this position relaxed with a gentle abdominal breathing, relieve the pressure on your knees but keep your hands around them. Relax your back, relax your shoulders, relax your arms.
8. Put your feet down first with bent knees, then stretch your legs down, your arms up — inhale — s t r e t c h.
9. Bring your arms down — exhale.

Relax.

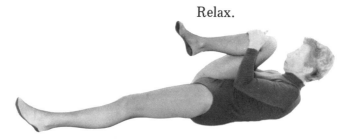

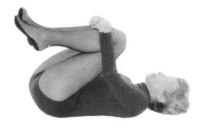

9TH WEEK.

WALK ON CEILING AND CROSSED LEGS.

To stretch and to strengthen the back, stomach and leg muscles. To stretch and to slim down the inner side of the thighs.

1. Lie on your back, bring your knees up to your chest.
2. Stretch your legs straight up and stretch your arms up in the air.
3. Keep your legs stretched and move them forward and backward about 2 feet apart, the same with your arms. *Slowly.*

About 10 X

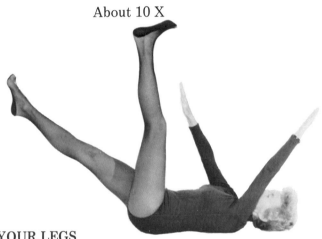

CROSSING YOUR LEGS.

1. Now hold legs and arms together up in the air.
2. Spread your legs and arms apart to the sides.
3. Cross your legs and cross your arms.
4. Spread legs and arms apart again. *Slowly. Not if pregnant.*

5 X

Watch your muscles carefully. You should only feel a gentle stretch in your inner thighs, not a strain.

R e l a x.

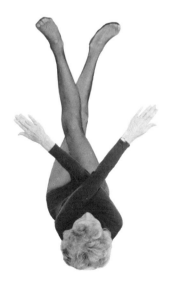

NECK RELAXING MOVEMENTS.

1. Sit cross-legged or on chair.
2. Slowly let your head go down, chin to chest.
3. Slowly raise your head and bring it back.

5 X

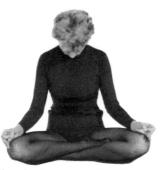
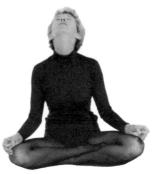

1. Slowly turn your head to your right side.
2. Slowly turn your head to your left side.

5 X

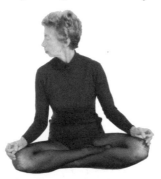
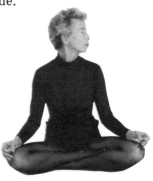

1. Slowly tilt your head toward your right shoulder.
2. Raise it up and tilt it slowly toward your left shoulder.

5 X

Stretch your legs and
relax your legs by
gently shaking
them.

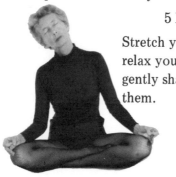
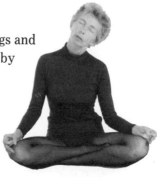

ROCK AND ROLL.

1. Sit up, bend your knees, feet on mat.
2. Clasp your hands gently together under your knees.
3. Put your chin to your chest.
4. Swing your legs up gently and roll back to your shoulderblades.
5. Swing your legs down and roll up — feet on mat.

10 X

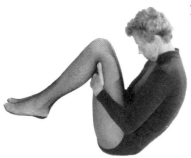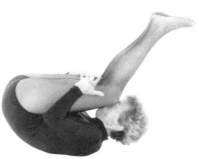

CROSS-LEGGED ROCK AND ROLL.

1. Sit up, cross your legs, hold on to your feet from the outside.
2. Lean back slightly, raise your feet about 10 inches up.
3. Stretch your arms to get your feet away from the body.
4. Slowly let yourself roll back to the back of your head — keep your knees bent.
5. Bring your feet to the crotch and let yourself roll up.

5 X

Each time try to do it more slowly than the time before.

Lie down and relax.

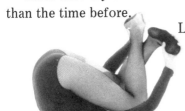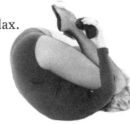

THE HALF SHOULDERSTAND.

1. Lie on your back, put your hands under your buttocks.
2. Slowly raise your legs and hips; carry the weight of your hips on your hands.
3. Hold this position relaxed with a gentle abdominal breathing. Direct your consciousness to your head; feel the blood circulating better in every part of your head. Hold 10-15 seconds.
4. Bring your feet slightly farther over your head.
5. Put your hands down on the mat close together.
6. Bend your knees and slowly roll your back down, bring your hips down and stretch your legs down.

   Lie there and relax.

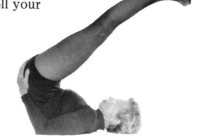

BACK RELAXING EXERCISE.

1. Lie on your back, bring your knees up high to your chest.
2. Put your hands on your knees, fingertips pointing toward your feet.
3. Slowly describe circles with your knees.

   5 X in each direction.

   Stretch your legs and relax.

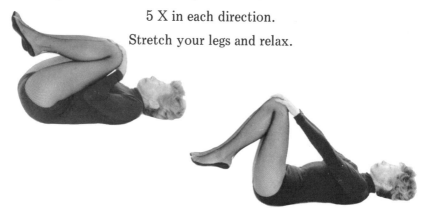

242

PLOW POSTURE AND KNEE TO EAR POSE
(OR KNEE TO FOREHEAD POSE.)

1. Lie on your back, put your hands under your buttocks, starting with palms down.
2. Slowly raise your legs and hips and keep going slowly farther back — as far as you can without feeling any strain. If you can touch your toes to the mat, hold the position with stretched legs for a few seconds.
3. Then bend your knees and put them on your forehead or put them down beside your ears.
4. Hold either position relaxed for 5-10 seconds, do a gentle abdominal breathing.
5. Then put your hands down on the mat close together, keep your knees bent and slowly roll your back down, bring your hips down and stretch you legs down.

2 X

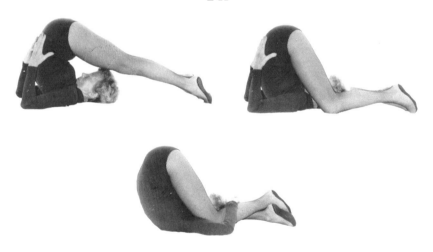

Lie down and relax.

9TH WEEK.

SIT UP AND ROLL DOWN.

To relax your back after the Plow Posture or the preparation for the Plow. Also to strengthen your abdominal muscles and to give you a nice flat tummy.

1. Lie on your back, bend your knees slightly, feet flat on the mat.
2. Raise your arms over your head.
3. Swing your arms up, roll your body up, bend forward relaxed over your bent knees.
4. Keep your arms beside your body and slowly roll your back down vertebra by vertebra, keep your chin to your chest to the last moment, roll your neck and head down.

3 X

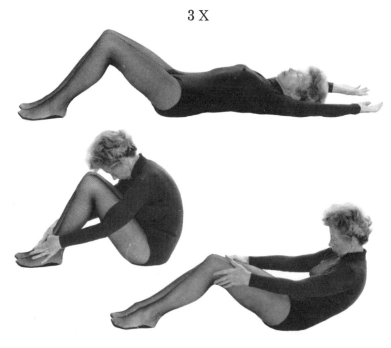

If you have trouble coming up this way, then sit up over your right side. Your muscles work this way also and do not get strained. In this exercise the rolling back is the more important part to relax your back muscles and to strengthen your abdominal muscles.

Now your back and neck are relaxed enough to go into the Straight Shoulderstand.

THE STRAIGHT SHOULDERSTAND.

The inverted position relieves pressure on your abdominal organs. The pressing of the chin to the chest (Chin lock) stops to a certain degree the blood circulation to the head. The blood circulation is increased in the front of the neck where the thyroid glands are located. Through the increased circulation they work better. Since the thyroid glands control the weight, bringing them back to good working order can regulate your weight. If you are too heavy you can lose some weight, or if you are too skinny you can gain some weight by practicing this exercise every day.

1. Lie on your back, put your hands under your buttocks, starting with palms down.
2. Slowly raise your legs and your hips, support your hips with your hands.
3. Now very slowly stretch your legs up straighter and slide your hands to your back, support your back well, elbows on mat. Hold for a few seconds if possible and comfortable.
4. To come down: *First lower your hips down,* slide your hands to your hips, your legs come down toward your face at the same time and you are in the Half Shoulderstand.
5. Bring your legs slightly farther over your head, put your hands down on the mat close together, bend your knees and slowly roll your back down, bring your hips down and stretch your legs down.

2 X

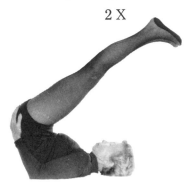

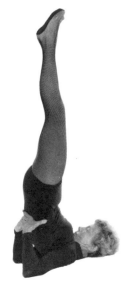

9TH WEEK.

BRIDGE POSTURE.

1. Lie on your back, arms relaxed alongside your body.
2. Bend your knees, feet on the mat slightly apart.
3. Slowly raise your hips while inhaling.
4. Lower your hips while exhaling, press your back down, draw your tummy in.

3 X

Lie down and relax.

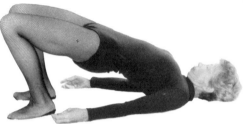

FORWARD BEND.

1. Sit up slowly over your right side and spread your legs apart.
2. Slowly raise your arms at your sides over your head while inhaling.
3. Bend down over your right leg while exhaling.
4. Slide your hands up your leg, raise your arms at your sides over your head while inhaling.
5. Bend down over your left leg while exhaling.

2 X

1. Bring your legs together, raise your arms at your sides while inhaling.
2. Bend down over both legs while exhaling.

2 X

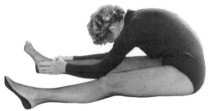 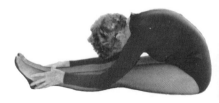

Relax your legs by shaking them gently.

9TH WEEK.

THE PLANE.

1. In the sitting position put your hands behind you.
2. Slowly raise your hips while inhaling, stretch your whole body, let your head go back. (Don't point your toes, keep your feet relaxed.)
3. Lower your hips while exhaling.

2 X

Relax your wrists, relax your arms, relax your legs by shaking them gently.

Lie down and relax.

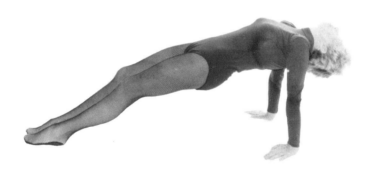

9TH WEEK.

BACK EXERCISE NO. 1.

1. Lie on your stomach, stretch your arms forward.
2. Keep stretching forward, close your eyes, direct your consciousness to your spine. Slowly raise your right arm, your left leg and your head while inhaling.
3. Slowly lower arm, leg and head while exhaling.
4. Slowly raise your left arm, your right leg and your head while inhaling.
5. Slowly lower your arm, leg and head while exhaling.

2 X

Put your hands under your chin and relax.

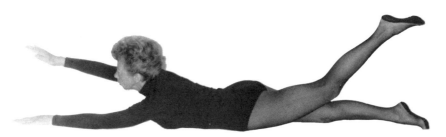

BACK EXERCISE NO. 2.

1. Lie on your stomach, arms alongside your body.
2. Slowly raise your upper body, your legs and arms while inhaling.
3. Slowly lower them while exhaling.

3 X

Put your hands under your chin and relax.

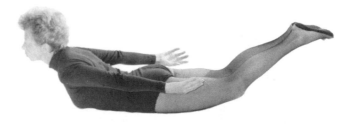

PREPARATION FOR COBRA POSTURE.

1. Lie on your stomach, put your hands under your shoulders, fingertips pointing toward each other.
2. Put your forehead on the mat.
3. Very slowly raise *your head* while inhaling.
4. Slowly lower your head while exhaling.

Direct your consciousness to the muscles in the middle part of your back.

If we practice the Cobra Posture alone (not during the Sun sequence, it is easier to hold the position with the fingers pointing to each other.

2 X

Relax.

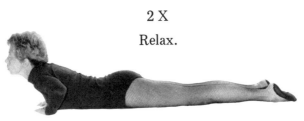

THE COBRA.

1. Lie on your stomach, put your hands under your shoulders, fingertips pointing toward each other.
2. Put your forehead on the mat, feet slightly apart.
3. During inhalation slowly raise your head, raise your chest, raise your upper body (pelvic area should stay on the mat, arms are slightly bent).
4. During exhalation slowly lower your body, roll your chest down, your head is the last part to come down.

2 X

Relax.

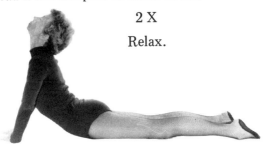

9TH WEEK.

YOGA MUDRA.

1. Sit back on your heels.
2. Raise your arms sideways over your head slowly while inhaling.
3. Slowly bend forward while exhaling. Keep sitting on your heels, put your hands behind your back, reach for your right wrist.
4. Put your head in the most comfortable position on the mat.
5. Hold the position and do a gentle abdominal breathing; feel your back muscles relax. Hold as long as you feel comfortable.
6. Slowly raise your body up. Get on your hands and knees, put your feet over to one side, sit down on the other side, stretch your legs, relax your legs, lie down and

r e l a x.

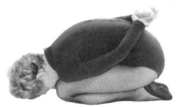

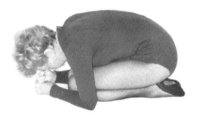

If you cannot yet sit comfortably on your heels, keep practicing The Foot Exercises every day a few times. You don't have to sit on the floor to practice them. When you sit on a chair cross your legs and work with one foot at a time. The more flexible your ankles become, the more comfortable you will feel sitting on your heels.

9TH WEEK.

CRAWLING. (On all fours around your living room.)

1. Get on your hands and knees.
2. Bring your right knee and your left hand forward.
3. Bring your left knee and your right hand forward.

Keep doing this and crawl around your living room 4 times, but only if you feel comfortable and relaxed.

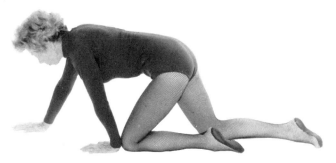

It is important that you always do the movement crosswise, that means right knee and left arm are moving forward and then left knee and right arm. If you have trouble doing it this way, watch it for a while. It is important to work properly on every muscle in your body and to strengthen them equally. It will come the right way when you are relaxed. I found that some children have problems doing it crosswise in the beginning. They are the ones who are not too well coordinated and their muscles are out of balance. After a short time of crawling activities, they start to move better in all their games and sports activities.

THE RELAXING POSTURE.

Close your eyes and lie in the most comfortable position. Arms slightly away from your body. Palms turned up. Shoulders relaxed.

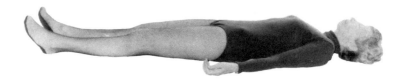

Relax your legs.
Relax your feet.
Relax your toes.
Relax your calves.
Relax your thighs.
Relax your stomach.
Relax your chest.
Relax your shoulders.
Relax your arms.
Relax your hands.
Relax your fingers.
Relax your neck.
Relax your head.
Relax your face.
Relax your mouth.
Relax your teeth.
Relax every muscle in your back.
Relax your whole body.
Relax completely.

Relax for 10 minutes. Then raise your arms over your head and s t r e t c h; roll on your left side and s t r e t c h; roll on your right side and s t r e t c h. Sit up over your right side.

Thank you, see you tomorrow.

SUMMARY

NINTH WEEK'S EXERCISES.

WARM-UPS.

1. Arm Swinging.   10 X
2. Knee Raising.   10 X
3. Side Bend.   3 X each side.
4. Arm Circles.   10 X
5. Shoulders Rolling. 5 X
6. Squatting Down.   4 X
7. Stretching Up.   2 X

YOGA EXERCISES.

1. The Salutation to the Sun. 2 X. Relax.
2. The 3 Parts of Breathing. 5 X each.
3. The Foot Exercises. 5 X each.
4. *The Complete Breath with Color.* 5 X
5. *The Leg Raising. (Variation.)* 2 X each. Relax.
6. Knee and Head Raising. 1 X each.
7. Walk on Ceiling and *Cross Legs.* 10 X and 5 X. Relax.
8. Neck Relaxing Movements.
9. Rock and Roll. 10 X
10. Cross-legged Rock and Roll. 5 X. Relax.
11. The Half Shoulderstand. Hold 10-15 seconds.
12. Back Relaxing Exercise. 5 X in each direction.
13. Plow Posture and Knee to Ear Pose. 2 X
14. *Sit Up and Roll Down.* 3 X. Relax.
15. The Straight Shoulderstand. 2 X. Relax.
16. Bridge Posture. 3 X. Relax.
17. Forward Bend. 2 X each.
18. The Plane. 2 X. Relax.
19. Back Exercise No. 1. 2 X each. Relax.
20. Back Exercise No. 2. 3 X. Relax.

9TH WEEK.

21. _Preparation for Cobra._ 2 X. Relax.
22. _Cobra._ 2 X
23. Yoga Mudra. 1 X
24. Crawling. (4 rounds in your living room.)
25. The Relaxing Posture.

TENTH WEEK'S EXERCISES.

Lie down and relax for a few minutes. Then sit up over your right side; stand up slowly and let's start with the Warm-up exercises.

WARM-UPS.

1.	Arm Swinging.	10 X
2.	Knee Raising.	10 X
3.	Side Bend.	3 X
4.	Arm Circles.	10 X
5.	Shoulders Rolling.	5 X
6.	Squatting Down.	4 X
7.	Stretching Up.	2 X

TENTH WEEK'S YOGA EXERCISES.

BALANCING EXERCISE NO. 6. DANCER'S POSE.

1. Stand on your right foot.
2. Raise your left leg and reach for your toes with your left hand.
3. Stretch your right arm straight up.
4. Slowly bring your right arm forward and raise your left leg.
5. Concentrate on one spot 3-4 feet in front of you.
6. Now slowly bring your leg higher up and stretch your arm straight up. Feel the gentle stretch in your back and your upper leg.
7. Slowly lower your arm and leg. Relax your legs, relax your shoulders.

Repeat on your left foot.

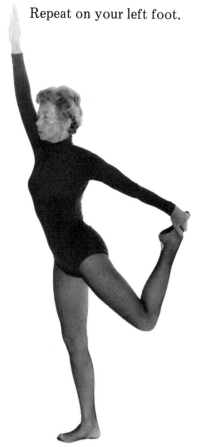

WIDE KNEE BEND AND SHIFT.

1. Put your feet wider apart than is comfortable.
2. Keep your feet parallel, toes pointing straight forward.
3. Bend your right knee, keep left leg stretched.
4. Come up, shift over and bend left knee.

10 X

1. Stay down and shift from side to side.

10 X

Relax your legs.

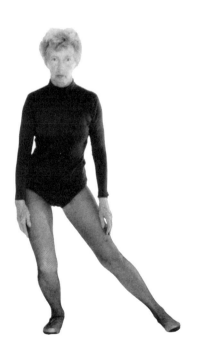

10TH WEEK.

TRIANGLE POSTURE.

1. Put your feet comfortably apart.
2. Raise your arms, palms up to shoulder height while inhaling.
3. Turn your right hand around, bend down to your right side, while exhaling. Hold the position with a gentle abdominal breathing 5-10 seconds.
4. Slowly raise your body up, turn your hands around while inhaling.
5. Bend down to your left side while exhaling. Hold the position about 5-10 seconds, do a gentle abdominal breathing.
6. Slowly raise your body up. Relax your legs.

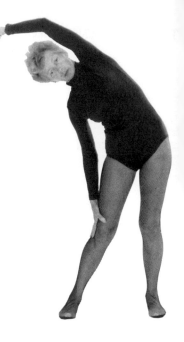

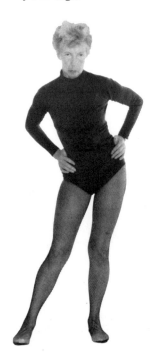

HIPROLLS.

1. Put your feet comfortably apart.
2. Put your hands on your hips.
3. Roll your hips around gently.

   10 X in each direction.

THE SALUTATION TO THE SUN. (SUN EXERCISE.)

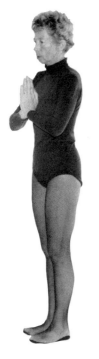

1. Put your hands to-
   gether in front of
   your chest.

2. Raise your arms
   over your head
   while inhaling,
   bend your head
   back gently.

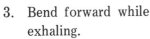

3. Bend forward while
   exhaling.

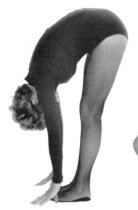

4. Put your hands down,
   stretch your right leg
   back, raise your head
   while inhaling.

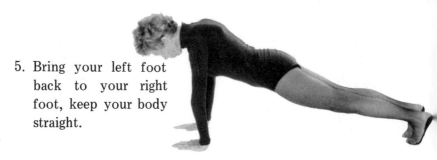

5. Bring your left foot back to your right foot, keep your body straight.

6. Put your knees down, lower your chest and your chin, exhale.

7. Put your hips down, stretch up to the Cobra while inhaling.

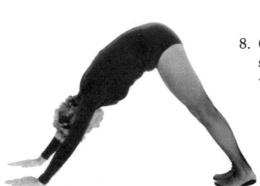

8. Curl in your toes, stretch up your hips while exhaling.

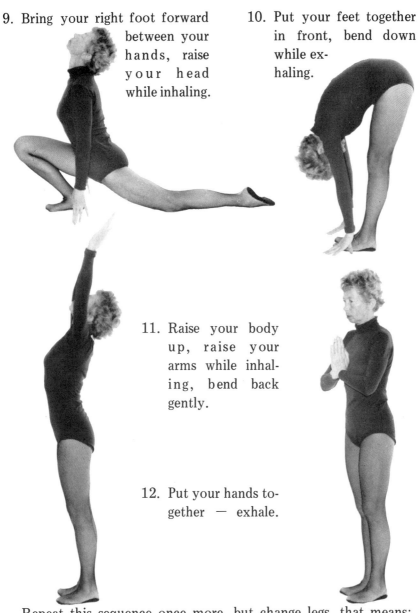

9. Bring your right foot forward between your hands, raise your head while inhaling.

10. Put your feet together in front, bend down while exhaling.

11. Raise your body up, raise your arms while inhaling, bend back gently.

12. Put your hands together — exhale.

Repeat this sequence once more, but change legs, that means:
In position 4 you stretch your left leg back,
in position 9 you bring your left foot forward.

Lie down and r e l a x.

261

10TH WEEK.

THE SUN BALANCE NO. 1.

To stretch and slim down your upper legs, to stretch the muscles in your chest, arms and shoulders. To raise your ribcage.

1. Sit up slowly over your right side and get on your hands and knees.
2. Put your right foot forward between your hands, put your whole weight on your right foot and stretch your right knee forward, stretch your left leg back. Stay down deep.
3. Slowly raise your arms in front over your head while inhaling. Bend back gently.
4. Slowly lower your arms while exhaling.
5. Bring your right knee back to your left knee, relax your legs by gently bouncing them up and down on your mat.

Repeat with your left foot in front.

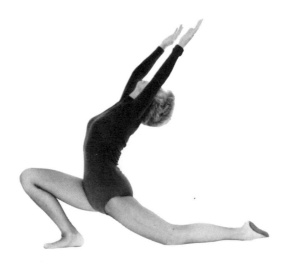

If you seem to lose your balance easily, try to stretch your leg back as far as you can; this way you have more surface to rest on. If you only rest on your knee bones it will be harder to balance.

262

10TH WEEK.

THE BREATHING EXERCISES.

THE ABDOMINAL BREATHING.

1. Sit in cross-legged position, put your hands on your tummy.
2. Draw your tummy in — exhale.
3. Let your tummy go out — inhale.
4. Draw your tummy in — exhale.

5 X

We have practiced the Abdominal Breathing now for several weeks. You should be ready for the next more advanced breathing exercise: "The Cleansing Breath" in sanskrit called "Kapalabhati." It is done only with the abdominal breathing. Instead of exhaling slowly we exhale fast by drawing in the abdominal muscles fast; they push fast against the diaphragm; it pushes fast against the lowest part of the lungs and the stale air or the carbon dioxide is pushed fast through the breathing passages, cleaning them out. The fast movement of the air through the breathing passages also increases the blood circulation in them and strengthens them. If practiced regularly this breathing exercise makes you practically immune to catching colds. If you have a cold when you start practicing it the first few times, it would be good to have a kleenex nearby. If you are pregnant you should not practice this breathing exercise, but practice all the other breathing exercises we have learned so far.

THE CLEANSING BREATH. KAPALABHATI.

1. Sit in cross-legged position.
2. We always start with an exhalation, so draw your tummy in — exhale.
3. Slowly let your tummy go out — inhale.
4. *Fast* draw your tummy in — exhale. It comes out like a sneeze. You help to a certain degree too, to push the air out, so make the sneeze an audible one, like you really want to clean out your nose.

5 X

5 X of this breath is called one round. After one round comes one complete breath and then the next round follows. Do two rounds when you practice it the first time.

When you have practiced two rounds for a few days you can add one more round, but never more than that.

After practicing it you will get a warm feeling in your chest, your throat and your face. It really increases the blood circulation in your breathing passages.

Caution: Use only the abdominal breathing for this Cleansing Breath. If you fill your lungs in the middle and the upper part, you cannot exhale all the carbon dioxide coming back during this fast short exhalation and you will get slightly dizzy or lightheaded. If that should happen, just lie down and relax and when you practice the next time watch it carefully that you use only your abdominal breathing for the inhalation.

THE LEG RAISING.

1. Lie completely relaxed, arms alongside your body.
2. Inhale — raise your right leg slowly, slide your hands up your leg, bring it gently closer toward your upper body.
3. Lower your right leg down while exhaling.
4. Inhale — raise your left leg slowly, slide your hands up your leg, bring it gently closer toward your upper body.
5. Lower your left leg slowly while exhaling.

2 X

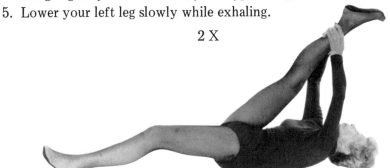

1. Put your hands under your buttocks, palms down.
2. Inhale — raise both legs slowly, slide your hands up your legs, bring them gently closer, don't raise your hips.
3. Put your hands under your buttocks again, lower your legs slowly while exhaling.

   Not for pregnant women.

2 X

KNEE AND HEAD RAISING.

1. Raise your arms over your head while inhaling — stretch.
2. Raise your right knee up to your chest, bring your hands and your head to your knee — exhale.
3. Put your head down, stretch your leg down, your arms up — inhale — stretch.
4. Raise your left knee up to your chest, bring your hands and your head to your knee — exhale.
5. Put your head down, stretch your leg down, your arms up — inhale — stretch.
6. Raise both knees up to your chest, bring your hands to your knees, press them down — exhale.
7. Hold this position relaxed — relieve the pressure on your knees, keep your hands around them. Breathe gently. Relax your back, relax your shoulders, relax your arms.
8. Put your feet down first, then stretch your legs down, your arms up — inhale — stretch.
9. Bring your arms down — exhale.

Relax.

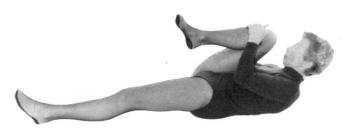

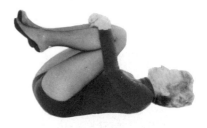

10TH WEEK.

NECK RELAXING MOVEMENTS.

1. Sit cross-legged.
2. Slowly let your head go down, chin to chest.
3. Slowly raise your head up and bring it back.

5 X

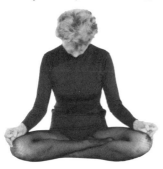 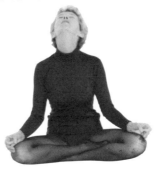

1. Slowly turn your head to your right side.
2. Slowly turn your head to your left side.

5 X

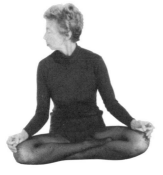 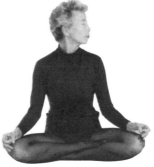

1. Slowly tilt your head toward your right shoulder.
2. Raise it up and tilt it slowly toward your left shoulder.

5 X

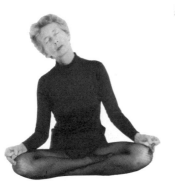 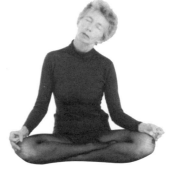

ROCK AND ROLL.

1. Sit up, bend your knees, feet on mat.
2. Clasp your hands gently together under your knees.
3. Put your chin to your chest.
4. Swing your legs up gently and roll back to your shoulderblades.
5. Swing your legs down and roll up — feet on mat. Direct your consciousness to your spine.

10 X

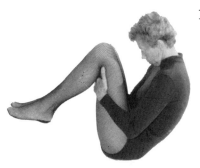
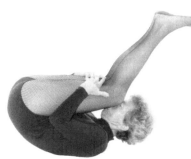

CROSS-LEGGED ROCK AND ROLL.

1. Sit up, cross your legs, hold on to your feet from the outside.
2. Lean back slightly, raise your feet about 10 inches.
3. Stretch your arms to get your feet away from the body.
4. Slowly let yourself roll back to the back of your head, keep your knees bent.
5. Bring your feet toward the crotch.
6. Let yourself roll up.

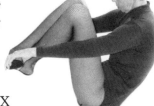

5 X

Lie down and relax.

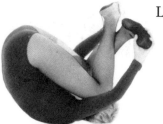
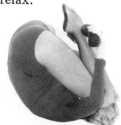

10TH WEEK.

THE HALF SHOULDERSTAND WITH BALANCE.

1. Lie on your back, put your hands under your buttocks, palms down.
2. Slowly raise your legs and hips; carry the weight of your hips on your hands.
3. Hold this position for a few seconds; do a gentle abdominal breathing.
4. Now raise your hips just a little bit higher and try to balance on your shoulderblades without help of your elbows.
5. Slide your hands up your legs and hold with stretched arms.
   Carry the weight of your legs on your arms.
   Hold a few seconds.
6. Slide your hands down to your hips, bring your feet slightly farther over your head. Put your hands down on the mat, close together.
7. Bend your knees and slowly roll your back down, bring your hips down and stretch your legs down.

   Relax.

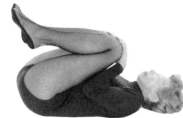

BACK RELAXING EXERCISE.

1. Lie on your back, bring your knees high up to your chest.
2. Put your hands on your knees, fingertips pointing toward your feet.
3. Slowly describe circles with your knees.

   5 X in each direction.

   Stretch your legs and relax.

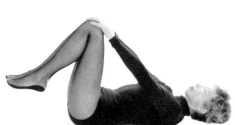

PLOW POSTURE AND KNEE TO EAR POSE
(OR KNEE TO FOREHEAD POSE).

1. Lie on your back, put your hands under your buttocks, starting with palms down.
2. Slowly raise your legs and hips, keep going *slowly* in the same spine bending movement farther back without feeling any strain. If you can touch your toes to the mat, hold the position with stretched legs for a few seconds. (Don't force them down.)
3. Then bend your knees and put them down on your forehead or put them down beside your ears. If your knees touch the mat, you can put your arms around your knees, but don't push them down.
4. Hold either position relaxed for 5-10 seconds.
5. Then put your hands on the mat close together, keep your knees bent and slowly roll your back down, bring your hips down and stretch your legs down.

Lie down and relax.

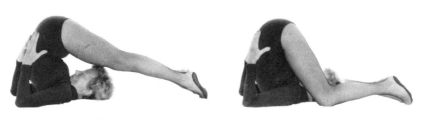

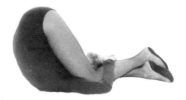

Repeat Back Relaxing Exercise before doing the Straight Shoulderstand.

10TH WEEK.

THE STRAIGHT SHOULDERSTAND.

1. Lie on your back, put your hands under your buttocks, palms down.
2. Slowly raise your legs and your hips and stretch up as straight as you can, support your back, elbows on the mat, close to body. If you feel comfortable and relaxed, hold the position for a few seconds, close your eyes, do a gentle abdominal breathing. But the moment you start feeling uncomfortable, come down slowly.
3. To come down: *First lower your hips*, slide your hands to your buttocks, your legs come down toward your face.
4. Put your hands on the mat, bend your knees and *slowly* roll your back down, bring your hips down and stretch your legs down. And r e l a x.

When we start holding any position longer, watch your body inside, become aware how your muscles feel. Never force yourself to hold the position longer than you can do it easily and relaxed.

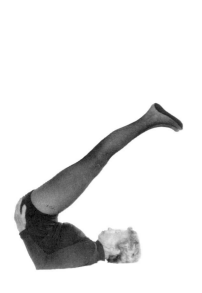 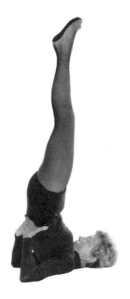

10TH WEEK.

BRIDGE POSTURE.

1. Lie on your back, arms relaxed alongside your body.
2. Bend your knees, feet on the mat slightly apart.
3. Slowly raise your hips while inhaling.
4. Lower your hips slowly while exhaling, press your back down, draw your tummy in.

3 X

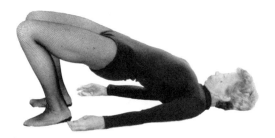

The Bridge Posture should always follow the Straight Shoulderstand to give the neck muscles time to relax in the normal position before we bend them in another direction. The opposite direction will be in the Fish Posture, we are going to learn today. The Fish Posture bends the neck back in the opposite direction from the Straight Shoulderstand. The muscles in the upper back are contracted, the muscles in the chest stretched. Read the instructions especially carefully before you start the posture.

10TH WEEK.

THE FISH POSTURE.

Limbers up and makes the neck and upper back more flexible. Stretches the front of the neck and prevents wrinkles and double chin. Develops a good posture and prevents dowager hump.

1. Sit up slowly over your right side.
2. Lean back on your elbows, keep legs stretched.
3. Raise your chest high up, let your head go back *slowly*.
4. Slide your arms forward until you rest on top of your head.
5. Keep your chest up high, keep your elbows on the mat for support. Do a gentle abdominal breathing.
6. To come out of it: Push down with your arms, raise your head up slightly. Lie down and relax.
7. Slowly turn your head from side to side to relax the muscles we just stretched.

2 X

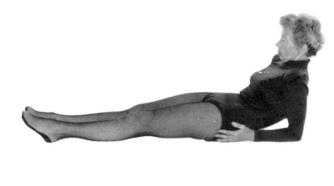

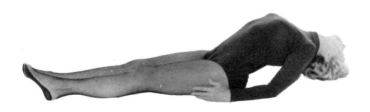

Before doing The Fish Posture read the following page.

When you do the Fish Posture the first time, do it very slowly, especially when you let your head go back; watch yourself carefully. If you should feel even only very slightly dizzy or lightheaded, *don't continue with the exercise.* Raise your head up and lie down and relax. But try it again the next day. In most cases this feeling disappears after a few days when the body gets used to this stretch. Only a few cases always have trouble with this posture and should not do it. These are people who also get carsick or seasick easily or have problems with the inner ear. Through practicing all the other Yoga exercises some of these problems could disappear.

People with a very long neck will feel uncomfortable or will feel a strain when raising the head coming out of the posture. They should only raise the head very slightly off the mat and then put it down. The Fish Posture is a beautiful exercise and after practicing it a few times you will love it. *Not during pregnancy or shortly after.*

10TH WEEK.

FORWARD BEND.

1. Sit up slowly over your right side and spread your legs apart.
2. Slowly raise your arms at your sides over your head while inhaling.
3. Bend down over your right leg while exhaling.

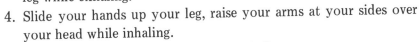

4. Slide your hands up your leg, raise your arms at your sides over your head while inhaling.
5. Bend down over your left leg while exhaling.

2 X

1. *Keep your legs apart,* raise your arms at your sides over your head while inhaling.
2. Bend down over the middle, reach for your feet or ankles while exhaling. Do it gently the first time. You don't have to bend all the way down, to get the benefits. Just as far as you can easily and relaxed.

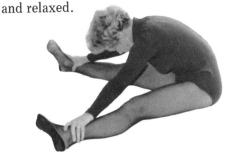

2 X

1. Bring your legs together, raise your arms at your sides over your head while inhaling.
2. Bend down over both legs while exhaling. Hold the position a few seconds with a gentle abdominal breathing.

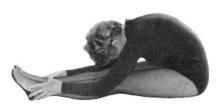

2 X

THE ALTERNATE LEG BEND.

1. In the sitting position spread your legs apart.
2. Put the sole of your left foot against the inside of your right thigh.
3. Raise your arms at your sides over your head while inhaling.
4. Bend slowly over your stretched leg while exhaling.

2 X

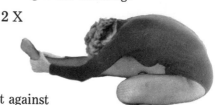

1. Spread your legs apart again.
2. Put the sole of your right foot against the inside of your left thigh.
3. Raise your arms at your sides over your head while inhaling.
4. Bend slowly over your stretched leg while exhaling.

2 X

Stretch your leg, relax your legs.

THE PLANE.

1. In the sitting position put your hands behind you.
2. Slowly raise your hips while inhaling; stretch your body, let your head go back.
3. Lower your hips down while exhaling.

2 X

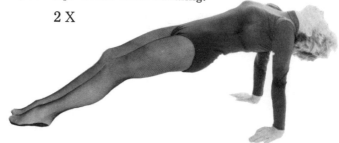

Be careful and don't stretch your toes down. To get your feet down, raise your hips higher up, but don't force it. It comes in time when your body gets stronger and more flexible.

Relax your wrists, relax your arms, relax your legs.

276

10TH WEEK.

THE HIPWALK.

To relax all the muscles in your body and to slim down buttocks, hips and upper legs.

1. Sit straight, legs stretched.
2. Raise your right hip up and push right leg forward.
3. Raise your left hip up and push left leg forward.
4. Let your hips do the walking, keep legs stretched. Swing your arms with the hip movement. Use your whole upper body, but do it relaxed. About 5 feet forward and 5 feet back.

Lie down and relax.

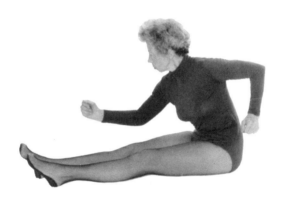

10TH WEEK.

CRAWLING. (On all fours around your living room.)

1. Get on your hands and knees.
2. Bring your right knee and your left hand forward.
3. Bring your left knee and your right hand forward. Keep doing this and crawl around your living room floor 4 times, but only if you feel comfortable and relaxed.

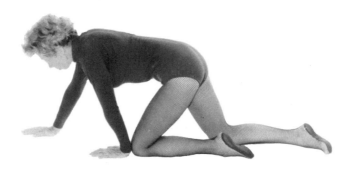

It is important that you always do the movement crosswise, that means right knee and left arm are moving forward and then left knee and right arm. If you have trouble doing it this way watch it for a while. It is important to work properly on every muscle in your body and to strengthen them equally. It will come the right way when you are relaxed. I found that some children have problems doing it crosswise in the beginning. They are the ones who are not too well coordinated and their muscles are out of balance. After a short time of crawling activities, they start to move better in all their games and sports activities.

THE RELAXING POSTURE.

Close your eyes and lie in the most comfortable position. Arms slightly away from your body.

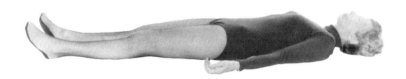

Relax your legs.
Relax your feet.
Relax your toes.
Relax your claves.
Relax your thighs.
Relax your stomach,
Relax your chest.
Relax your shoulders.
Relax your arms.
Relax your hands.
Relax your fingers.
Relax your neck.
Relax your head.
Relax your face.
Relax your mouth.
Relax your teeth.
Relax every muscle in your back.
Relax your whole body.
Relax completely.

Relax for 10 minutes. Then raise your arms over your head and s t r e t c h. Roll on your left side and s t r e t c h, roll on your right side and s t r e c h. Sit up over your right side.

Thank you, see you tomorrow.

10TH WEEK.

SUMMARY

TENTH WEEK'S EXERCISES.

WARM-UPS.

1. Arm Swinging.   10 X
2. Knee Raising.   10 X
3. Side Bend.   3 X each side.
4. Arm Circles.   10 X
5. Shoulders Rolling.   5 X
6. Squatting Down.   4 X
7. Stretching Up.   2 X

YOGA EXERCISES.

1. Balancing Exercise No. 6. Dancer's Pose. 1 X each leg.
2. Wide Knee Bend and Shift. 10 X each.
3. Triangle Posture. 1 X to each side.
4. Hiprolls. 10 X in each direction.
5. The Salutation to the Sun. 2 X. Relax.
6. *The Sun Balance No. 1.* 2 X. Relax.
7. The Abdominal Breathing. 5 X
8. *The Cleansing Breath.* 10 X (2 rounds.)
9. The Leg Raising. 2 X each. Relax.
10. Knee and Head Raising. 1 X each. Relax.
11. Neck Relaxing Movements. 5 X each.
12. Rock and Roll. 10 X
13. Cross-legged Rock and Roll. 5 X. Lie down and relax.
14. The Half Shoulderstand with Balance. 1 X
15. Back Relaxing Exercise. 5 X in each direction.
16. Plow Posture and Knee to Ear Pose or Knee to Forehead Pose. Relax.
17. Back Relaxing Exercise.
18. The Straight Shoulderstand. Relax.
19. The Bridge Posture. 3 X. Relax.
20. *The Fish Posture.* 2 X. Relax.

21. Forward Bend. 2 X each.
22. The Alternate Leg Bend. 2 X each.
23. The Plane with Hips Higher. 2 X. Relax.
24. *The Hipwalk.* Relax.
25. Crawling. (4 rounds.)
26. The Relaxing Posture.

SUMMARY OF THE 10 WEEKS COURSE.

FIRST WEEK:
WARM-UPS
Arm Swinging
Knee Raising
Side Bend
Arm Circles
Shoulders Rolling
Squatting Down
Stretch Up

YOGA EXERCISES:
Balancing #1
Wide Knee Bend and Shift
Triangle
Hiprolls
Leg Raising
Knee and Head Raising
Both Knees Up
Neck Movements
Rock and Roll
Half Shoulderstand
Bridge Posture
Relaxing Posture

SECOND WEEK:
WARM-UPS:
Arm Swinging
Knee Raising
Side Bend
Arm Circles
Shoulders Rolling
Squatting Down
Stretch Up

YOGA EXERCISES:
Balancing #1
Balancing #2
Wide Knee Bend and Shift
Triangle
Hiprolls
Abdominal Breathing
Middle or Ribcage Breathing
Upper or Chest Breathing
Leg Raising
Knee and Head Raising
Neck Movements
Rock and Roll
Half Shoulderstand
Bridge
Forward Bend
Alternate Leg Bend
Plane
Relaxing Posture

THIRD WEEK:
WARM-UPS:
YOGA EXERCISES:
Balancing #2
Wide Knee Bend and Shift
Triangle Posture
Hiprolls
Abdominal Breathing
Middle Breathing
Upper Breathing
Foot Exercises
The Complete Breath
The Leg Raising

Knee and Head Raising
Neck Movements
Rock and Roll
Half Shoulderstand
Bridge Posture
Forward Bend
Alternate Leg Bend
The Plane
Spinal Twist 1. Version
Push Ups
Wall Push Ups
Yoga Mudra
Relaxing Posture

FOURTH WEEK:
WARM-UPS:
YOGA EXERCISES:
Balancing #2
Wide Knee Bend and Shift
Triangle Posture
Hiprolls
Prep. for Sun Exercise:
　Upper Leg Stretch
　Hamstring Stretch
The 3 Parts of Breathing
Foot Exercises
Complete Breath
Leg Raising
Knee and Head Raising
Knees Over
Neck Movements
Rock and Roll
Cross-legged Rock and Roll
The Half Shoulderstand
Back Relaxing Exercise

Knee to Forhead Pose
Bridge Posture
Forward Bend
Spinal Twist 2. Verson
Back Exercises
Limbering Up Knees and Feet
Push Ups
Yoga Mudra
Relaxing Posture

FIFTH WEEK:
WARM-UPS:
YOGA EXERCISES:
Balancing #2
Wide Knee Bend and Shift
Triangle Posture
Hiprolls
Armstretch
Prep. for Sun Exercise:
　Upper Leg Stretch
　Hamstring Stretch
The 3 Parts of Breathing
Foot Exercises
The Complete Breath
The Leg Raising
Knee and Head Raising
Leg Up and Down
Neck Movements
Rock and Roll
Cross-legged Rock and Roll
The Half Shoulderstand
Back Relaxing Exercise
Knee to Forehead Pose
Bridge Posture
Forward Bend

Rest of an Animal
Crawling
The Relaxing Posture

SIXTH WEEK:
WARM-UPS:
YOGA EXERCISES:
Balancing Ex. #3
Wide Knee Bend and Shift
Triangle Posture
Hiprolls
Armstretch
Prep. for Sun Exercise
    Upper Leg Stretch
    Hamstring Stretch
    The Step Forward
The 3 Parts of Breathing
Foot Exercises
The Complete Breath
Leg Raising
Knee and Head Raising
Both Legs Down Slowly
Neck Movements
Rock and Roll
Cross-legged Rock and Roll
The Half Shoulderstand
Back Relaxing Exercise
Knee to Forehead Pose
Bridge Posture
Forward Bend
Back Exercise #1
Back Exercise #2
Preparation for Cobra Posture
The Cobra Posture
Yoga Mudra

Crawling
The Relaxing Posture

SEVENTH WEEK:
WARM-UPS:
YOGA EXERCISES:
Balancing Ex. #4
    (Dancer's Pose 1. Version)
Wide Knee Bend and Shift
Triangle Posture
Hiprolls
Prep. for Sun Exercise
    Upper leg Stretch
    Hamstring Stretch
    The Step Forward
    The 8 Point Touch
The Salutation to the Sun
    (Sun Exercise)
The 3 Parts of Breathing
Foot Exercises
The Complete Breath
Leg Raising
Knee and Head Raising
Walk on Ceiling
Neck Movements
Rock and Roll
Cross-legged Rock and Roll
The Half Shoulderstand
Back Relaxing Exercise
Knee to Forehead Pose
Sit Up and Roll Down
Straight Shoulderstand
Bridge Posture
Crawling
The Relaxing Pose

EIGHTH WEEK:
WARM-UPS:
YOGA EXERCISES:

Balancing Ex. #5
   (Dancer's Pose 2. Version)
Wide Knee Bend and Shift
Triangle Posture
Hiprolls
Armstretch
Armstretch Variation
The Salutation to the Sun
The 3 Parts of Breathing
Foot Exercises
The Complete Breath
Leg Raising
Knee and Head Raising
Leg Over
Neck Movements
Rock and Roll
Cross-legged Rock and Roll
The Half Shoulderstand with Balance
Back Relaxing Exercise
Knee to Forehead Pose
Plow Posture and Knee to Ear Pose
Bridge Posture
Forward Bend
The Alternate Leg Bend
The Plane
The Spinal Twist 3. Version
Catstretch #1
Crawling
The Relaxing Posture

NINTH WEEK:
WARM-UPS:
YOGA EXERCISES:

The Salutation to the Sun
The 3 Parts of Breathing
Foot Exercises
The Complete Breath
   with Color
Leg Raising
Knee and Head Raising
Walk on Ceiling
   and Cross Legs
Neck Movements
Rock and Roll
Cross-legged Rock and Roll
The Half Shoulderstand
Back Relaxing Exercise
Plow Posture
   and Knee to Ear
   or to Forehead Pose
Sit Up and Roll Down
The Straight Shoulderstand
Bridge Posture
Forward Bend
The Plane
Back Exercise #1
Back Exercise #2
Preparation for Cobra
Cobra
Yoga Mudra
Crawling
The Relaxing Posture

TENTH WEEK:

WARM-UPS:

YOGA EXERCISES:

Balancing Ex. #5
   (Dancer's Pose)
Wide Knee Bend and Shift
Triangle Posture
Hiprolls
The Salutation to the Sun
The Sun Balance #1
The Abdominal Breathing
The Cleansing Breath
   (Kapalabhati)
Leg Raising
Knee and Head Raising
Neck Movements
Rock and Roll
Cross-legged Rock and Roll
The Half Shoulderstand
   with Balance
Back Relaxing Exercise
Plow Posture and Knee to
   Ear or Forehead Pose
Back Relaxing Exercise
The Straight Shoulderstand
Bridge Posture
The Fish Posture
Forward Bend
The Alternate Leg Bend
The Plane
The Hipwalk
Crawling
The Relaxing Posture
Jogging

I hope you will feel a distinct improvement in your well-being after practicing Yoga exercises for 10 weeks. If you did it regularly or almost regularly you will feel better. Only one thing Yoga does not do for your body: It does not work on your cardio-vascular system. To increase your cardio-vascular output, you should do some activity which gets your pulse beat up to 130 beats per minute when you are over thirty years of age and to 150 beats per minute when you are under 30. It should be an activity which lasts at least 20-30 minutes to get the training or endurance effect.

During Yoga practice sessions you learn how to breathe. In your endurance activity you can use this ability. But before you start any endurance program have a check-up with your doctor. If everything is all right and he cannot find anything wrong with you, you can start with your program.

The best activity to start with is walking; walk in your neighborhood, join a hiking club, walk in the nearest park or on the beach, but do it regularly, not only once a year.

After walking for some weeks or months, you can try to jog for a short stretch during your walk. If you liked it and it felt good, jog a little bit longer the next time. Always walk afterwards again to slow down your heart beat, do not sit down or even lie down after jogging. The most important part of jogging is the breathing rhythm.

You have to get enough oxygen into your body and have to get the carbon dioxide out. I found an easy way to breathe and also a very efficient way is the following method:

You exhale through your mouth with the sound "Ha" twice with two steps. You inhale through your nose with two steps, also two times. It goes: exhale-step, exhale-step, inhale-step, inhale-step. The amazing thing is, you never get out of breath when you jog. Don't run. Jogging is a very slow, lazy trot. You hardly lift your feet, just let them fall forward. Come down on your whole foot, do not jog on the ball of your foot, this can give you very sore calves.

Wear comfortable shoes and warm clothes, if it is cold outside. Shorts and shirt, if it is warm. Try to find some trails in the woods or along the beach or in a park, do not jog on the road where cars are traveling; it is too dangerous and you are inhaling the exhaust fumes (carbon monoxide, sulphur oxide, lead, etc.)

If you are jogging in the gym, alternate walking with jogging until you feel strong enough to jog all the time. Always watch your body and take your pulse regularly.

Another good endurance activity is swimming. Start slowly with a few lengths of the pool and work up to ¼ of a mile or even ½ a mile.

With any one, or all of these activities and Yoga you can keep your body healthy and flexible until old age and really enjoy it.

3 YOGA EXERCISE RECORDS

"Yoga For Beginners"
"Yoga For Intermediates"
"Yoga for Advanced"

Spoken and demonstrated by Ruth Bender
Internationally known Physical Education and Yoga Teacher

"... they are the best Yoga records I have heard, you really can practice every day with them. They are just great!"

"... it is like being in one of Ruth Bender's classes!"

".... with her soothing voice I can relax completely!"

".... on this rainy Sunday the whole family had a marvelous time working out with these records!"

".... and even my husband is now starting and doing the exercises with me!"

These are some of the comments you can hear about Ruth Bender's records.

What can Yoga exercises do for you?

... trim and firm your figure
... normalize your weight
... teach you to relax and relieve tension
... acquire energy, overcome fatigue
They make you feel better from day to day.

It is the most beautiful, scientifically worked out exercise system to bring your body to good health and to good physical condition slowly and gently without strain or pain, without getting exhausted or tired.

Yoga exercises are for every physical condition and for every age for men, women and children.

Take the first step on the path of Yoga and order your record today.

Now also available on cassettes.